Basic Science & Clinical Applications
MEDICAL CANNABIS
What Clinicians Need to Know and Why

Dr Greg Smith

BASIC SCIENCE & CLINICAL APPLICATIONS

MEDICAL CANNABIS

WHAT CLINICIANS NEED TO KNOW AND WHY

GREGORY L. SMITH, MD, MPH

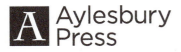

Aylesbury Press

8 West Street
Beverly Farms, MA 01915
www.aylesburypress.com

First Edition, 2016

ISBN 978-1-883595-72-2

Library of Congress Cataloging-in-Publication Data

Names: Smith, Gregory L., author.
Title: Medical cannabis : basic science & clinical applications : what
    clinicians need to know and why / Gregory L. Smith.
Description: Beverly Farms, MA : OEM Press, 2016. | Includes biblio-
    graphical references and index.
Identifiers: LCCN 2015049039 (print) | LCCN 2015050102 (ebook) |
    ISBN 9781883595722 (pbk.) | ISBN 9781883595739 (E-book)
Subjects: | MESH: Medical Marijuana | Cannabis
Classification: LCC RM666.C266 (print) | LCC RM666.C266 (ebook) | NLM
    WB 925 | DDC 615.7/827--dc23
LC record available at http://lccn.loc.gov/2015049039

Cover Design: Ellen Weinberger
Interior Design & Production: Matt Mayerchak, Cia Boynton
Printed in the United States of America

Aylesbury Press is an imprint of OEM Health Information, Inc.

Questions or comments regarding this book should be directed to:

Aylesbury Press
8 West Street
Beverly Farms, MA 01915-2226
(978) 921-7300
www.aylesburypress.com

10 9 8 7 6 5 4 3

To Dr. George and Patricia Smith, my thoughtful and caring parents, loving and considerate partners, and role models for many.

Notices

The author and the publisher have made every effort to ensure the accuracy and appropriateness of the drug dosages presented in this textbook. The medications described do not necessarily have specific approval by the Food and Drug Administration for the diseases and dosages for which they are recommended. It is the responsibility of practitioners to make diagnoses, to determine dosages, and the best treatment for each patient relying on their own experience and knowledge of their patients. Because the legal and regulatory environment is constantly evolving, readers are encouraged to confirm the information contained herein with other sources. In particular, readers are encouraged to comply with all applicable local, state, and Federal laws. The author and the publisher do not provide legal advice and readers are encouraged to consult a professional advisor for such advice. Neither the author nor the publisher warrants the information herein is in every aspect accurate or complete, and they disclaim all responsibility for any errors or omissions, liability, loss, injury, or damage incurred as a consequence, directly or indirectly, of the use and application of any of the contents of this volume.

Contents

Appendices

Preface

In the months after medical marijuana (cannabis) is legalized in your state, you notice that your patients are asking more and more questions about it. What type of cannabis? What conditions? What is THC versus CBD? What are the side-effects? Is it addictive? How is it prescribed?

What do you do? Read this concise, up-to-date and very informative book! As a recent *New York Times* article on medical cannabis implies, "It is not going away."

The fact that, at the time of this book's publication, medical cannabis is legal in a number of states but illegal at a federal level, is confusing. There is also confusion about dosing and which conditions respond to cannabis, adding to the uncertainty of the efficacy and safety of cannabis as medicine. As a result, most clinicians in the medical community are poorly informed and thus skeptical about medical cannabis.

This ambivalence toward medical cannabis was demonstrated by results of a 2013 survey of 520 family physicians in Colorado. Most of the physicians agreed that cannabis had significant mental and physical health risks. Only 19 percent of physicians believed that medical cannabis should be recommended for medical purposes. However, 80 percent agreed that information on it should be incorporated into medical school and residency education, and 92 percent agreed that it should be a topic covered in continuing medical education (CME) for practicing physicians. In short, most clinicians feel that cannabis is probably an effective medication, but the limited clinical research on conditions for which it is efficacious, as well as on scientifically-validated dosing, render it not yet ready for "prime time."

Many clinicians continue to hold old misconceptions about the addictive risk of medical cannabis, or they feel that the majority of persons using cannabis are doing so for recreational purposes under the guise of medicinal use. Many also have limited experience with a medication that comes as plant material, and they have minimal education on the active ingredients and the means of recommending medical cannabis to patients and managing these patients.

In addition to these realities, most of the health benefits, dosing, formulations, and routes of administration (delivery) for the target conditions are not supported by high-quality randomized, controlled trials, and the state-sanctioned medical conditions for which medical cannabis can be used are often based on public outcry, politics, and pseudoscience.[1]

Cannabis has a long and noble ancient history of medicinal use. However, the complex legal history and the association of cannabis with the euphoric effects from delta-9-tetrahydrocannabinol (THC) and its reputation as a "gateway drug," as well as its exaggerated association with "reefer madness," have made most clinicians wary of recommending cannabis for treatment. Clearly, the relatively recent discovery of the endocannabinoid system (ECS) in the brain and body and the plethora of new high-quality research into the effects of cannabis that are now underway, make medical cannabis an important and necessary part of a complete medical education.

Up to now there has been no serious textbook for training clinicians about the use, efficacy, and monitoring of medical cannabis. The books that have been published tend to have an overly simplistic, quasi-clinical approach, usually without a solid basic-science background or a clear, rational clinical approach.

The objective of this book is to provide the basic science and clinical information necessary to make the practicing primary care physician feel comfortable answering questions about cannabis as well as recommending it as a medication.

ACKNOWLEDGMENTS

I am grateful to Developmental Editor Kathleen O'Brien for her editorial advice and guidance with the early drafts of my manuscript. Alexis Rautio, Editorial Director at OEM Health Information, Inc., has worked tirelessly to bring this work to completion under a tight schedule. A special thank you to both of them for their support and encouragement—without them this book would not be a reality. Finally, I want to especially thank Kayla Stone, my indispensable administrative assistant. GLS

Terminology

2-arachidonoylglycerol (2-AG) An endogenous fatty acid neurotransmitter. It is a ligand of CB1 and present in higher levels in the central nervous system (CNS).

Anandamide (AEA) An endogenous fatty acid neurotransmitter. It is a ligand of CB1 and present in higher levels in the body.

Biosynthetic Cannabinoids Cannabinoid compounds that are manufactured with the use of enzymes that catalyze a series of chemical reactions to produce complex molecules from more simple molecules.

Cannabidiol (CBD) One of the most abundant cannabinoids in cannabis. It has no psychoactive effects.

Cannabinoid A substance that binds with the ECS receptors. There are two types of cannabinoids: phytocannabinoids, derived from plants; and endocannabinoids, that are endogenous to the body.

Cannabis The plant or plant material that is used for medicinal purposes or as a recreational drug.

Cannabis Dependence Syndrome A relatively mild condition, associated with withdrawal symptoms of dysphoria, disturbed sleep, gastrointestinal symptoms, and decreased appetite. In addition there is continued use of cannabis even though the person perceives continued use as problematic.

Cannabis Edibles Food items, candies, or beverages that are infused with specific doses of cannabinoids.

Cannabis Oil An oily cannabis product made through a variety of extraction processes and solvents. It is a highly concentrated form of cannabinoids.

Cannabis sativa I. The "I" stands for *indica*. One of the subspecies of the *Cannabis sativa*. It is a short bush, with broad leaves. It is known for having higher levels of THC compared to the amount of CBD.

Cannabis sativa S. The "S" stands for sativa. One of the subspecies of *Cannabis sativa*. It is tall with thin leaves. It is known for having higher levels of CBD compared to the amount of THC. Hemp is a strain of *Cannabis sativa S.*

Cannabis Tincture A liquid cannabis product made through extraction processes using either alcohol or glycerin.

Cesamet An FDA approved medication. The active ingredient is a synthetic analogue of delta-9-THC called nabilone.

Charlotte's Web A cultivar of *Cannabis sativa L.* with very low-THC and high levels of CBD used for intractable pediatric seizures.

Cytochrome P450 System (CYP) A system, principally in the liver, that catalyzes the metabolism of potential toxic compounds via several different types of reactions.

Dravet Syndrome A rare genetic epileptic encephalopathy marked by very frequent seizures in childhood.

Endocannabinoid Deficiency An unconfirmed medical condition that is caused by producing too little endogenous cannabinoids.

Endocannabinoid System (ECS) The innate neuromodulatory system in the brain and body that has cannabinoid receptors, agonists and antagonists, and enzymes of degradation.

ECS Receptors (CB1 and CB2) These are the designations for cannabinoid receptors found on cells throughout the brain and body.

Entourage Effect The synergistic effects associated with cannabinoids and terpenes.

Epidiolex A pharmaceutical grade medication, comprised of an extract of cannabis, which is very high in CBD and has no THC.

G protein-coupled receptor 55 (GPR55) A putative cannabinoid receptor. It may be designated CB3 in the near future.

Hashish A cannabis product comprised of compressed resin glands (trichomes).

Hemp Refers to industrial grade cannabis sativa plants and is very low in THC.

Marinol An FDA approved medication. The active ingredient is a synthetic analogue of delta-9-THC called dronabinol.

Palmitoylethanolamide (PEA) An endogenous fatty acid neurotransmitter. It is a ligand of GPR55.

Pharmacogenetics The study of individual variation in the genetic sequence related to drug response.

Phytocannabinoids Plant-based compounds that are analogues of endocannabinoids and that bind with ECS receptors.

Potency Determined by the percent of the plant material that is THC and THCa combined.

Routes of Administration Oral, topical, nasal, ingestion, inhalation, or injection are all means to administer a drug or medicine.

Sativex A pharmaceutical grade medication, comprised of two different extracts of cannabis, that are combined to provide approximately 1:1 THC:CBD ratio and dispensed for oromucosal absorption.

Synthetic Cannabinoids Cannabinoid compounds that are manufactured using chemical processes.

Terpenes Aromatic compounds with specific fragrances that are ubiquitous in the plant world. Dozens of different terpenes are found in cannabis.

Tetrahydrocannabinol (THC) A naturally occurring analogue of Anandamide and the most psychoactive cannabinoid in cannabis. There are two THCs: delta-9-THC, the most psychoactive; and delta-8-THC, which is very much like delta-9-THC but about 25 percent less psychoactive.

Transient Receptor Potential Vanilloid Receptor 1 (TRPV-1) A capsaicin receptor. It is involved with regulation of body temperature and heat nociception.

Trichomes Colorful crystalline structures that give the pungent aroma and often vivid variety of colors to the cannabis bud.

Vaporization The use of specific temperatures to convert a substance from a liquid to a gaseous state.

Why a Book for Clinicians on Medical Cannabis?

Since enactment of laws in dozens of states where medical cannabis is now legal, the few clinicians who currently recommend cannabis for medicinal use often write recommendation letters to almost everyone who asks. This is usually written after only a cursory physical examination and the payment of a cash fee. Many of the cannabis dispensaries visited by the author over the years have a comical, almost circus-like atmosphere. Over the years the concept of medical cannabis has been co-opted and viewed as only a means to bypass laws that

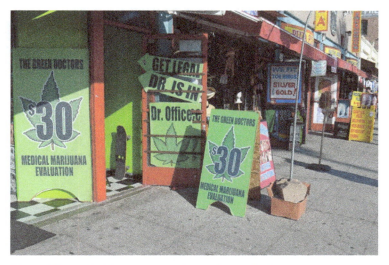

Medical Cannabis Dispensary in Venice Beach, California

prevent it from being used for recreational purposes. This medical marijuana/cannabis "circus" of the past needs to end!

Current Status of Medical Cannabis Use

APPLICATIONS FOR REGISTRATION
Data on medical cannabis use in Arizona between April and October 2011 showed that of 14,925 applicants for medical cannabis registration, only 7 were denied.

The most recent data from the 23 states and the District of Columbia, where medical cannabis is now legal, show that there are approximately 1.2 million legal users of medical cannabis, about 7 patients per 1,000 state residents. However, this number is growing rapidly.

See http://medicalmarijuana.procon.org/view.resource.php?resourceID=005889

INVOLVEMENT OF CLINICIANS AND DISPENSARIES
Because of the jaundiced and often unprofessional approach to medical cannabis, the majority of physicians in states where it is legal do not want to recommend it to patients or be associated with it in any way. In Colorado, where it has been legal for 15 years, only 10 percent of physicians have ever recommended it. Clinicians who do recommend medical cannabis usually take a passive, background role after writing a recommendation letter, infrequently monitoring patients for the drug's efficacy and adverse reactions.

Over the decades, the staff working at medical cannabis dispensaries have taken on an active role by helping the patients determine the best format for the medication (e.g., strains of flower bud, tinctures, edibles, vaporizers). However, the staff has little formal, standardized training or continuing education, and they rarely conduct any quality assurance programs or evidence-based medical documentation.

RESEARCH STUDIES
After President Nixon's "War on Drugs" was initiated in the 1970s, cannabis was categorized as a Schedule I narcotic—that is, to have "no currently accepted medical use and a high risk for addiction." This has resulted in four decades of almost no National Institutes of Health (NIH)-funded research on the

medicinal effects of cannabis. However, since medical cannabis started to become legal in the United States (and the world) there has been an abundance of new clinical literature on its effects. Previously, much of the clinical literature came from Europe and Israel, where it is less strictly controlled and where a variety of patented pharmacologic preparations of THC and/or CBD are available to clinicians.

| *High-quality studies are finally being published.*

In the early 1990s the endogenous cannabinoid system (ECS) was discovered. The ECS is an innate neuromodulatory system with cannabinoid receptors in the brain and throughout the body that affect a wide variety of psychoactive and physiologic processes. The discovery of the ECS has dramatically changed how plant-based cannabinoids are viewed by scientists; many now see them as legitimate and potent pharmaceutical agents.

STATE MEDICAL BOARDS

Unfortunately, the various state medical boards around the country, as well as the American Medical Association (AMA), have taken a somewhat hostile approach to the passage of medical cannabis laws. This lack of recognition or support has significantly hindered the development of training and certification programs for clinicians. Even the half-hearted attempt by the state of Florida to legalize medical cannabis resulted in legalizing only very low-level THC cannabis strains (cultivars) and the state required a burdensome 8-hour continuing medical education (CME) course focused solely on low-THC high-CBD cannabis. A clinician completing this $1,000 course gets a very limited education on THC and, in essence, doesn't gain clinical skills on the medicinal use of cannabis.

Nonetheless, clinicians are going to be bombarded with requests and questions about medical cannabis. The need for educated and experienced clinicians will increase exponentially if, as expected, the federal government moves cannabis from Schedule I of the Controlled Substances Act (CSA) to Schedule II, making it much more freely and easily available to use as a medication.

The negative view held by some states and some clinicians regarding the use of cannabis as medicine is often shared by federal agencies such as the National Institutes of Health (NIH). This negativity appears to be based on anachronistic views of "pot-smoking hippies" who try to circumvent the law to obtain medical cannabis for recreational use. To be fair, some of the excesses and circus-like atmosphere seen in California and Colorado dispensaries don't help mitigate this perception.

MEDICAL EDUCATION

Another reason for the dearth of clinicians actively "recommending" medical cannabis is a lack of formal training on this rapidly evolving subject. The clinician often feels inadequately educated on the topic and inept in the practical use of cannabis as medicine.

The author contacted all of the medical schools in the United States and Canada to request that they submit answers to several survey questions. The survey revealed that only about 25 percent of medical schools were providing education on the use of medical cannabis. In almost all schools that did provide some education, it amounted to only 1–4 hours of introductory education.

On a more promising note, many of the states that have legalized medical cannabis are requiring 4 or more hours of formal Category I CME on the topic. The components of this CME are usually detailed in the medical board rules.

MEDICAL VERSUS RECREATIONAL CANNABIS

Medical cannabis first became available in the United States in 1996, after California's Proposition 215 was enacted as state law. Since then, other states have legalized medical cannabis in a variety of complex and often inconsistent ways. Four states have legalized cannabis for recreational use, and it is expected that all of the states will eventually legalize medical, and perhaps recreational, cannabis as the "dominoes fall" over the next decade. In the states that already have legalized cannabis for both medical and recreational use, the two markets for cannabis operate independently of each other.

REGULATIONS AND RESTRICTIONS

There is a hodgepodge of regulations, requirements, and restrictions on how medical cannabis is grown and distributed. There are some basic similarities from state to state on how it is "prescribed" by physicians. The word "prescribed" is intentionally in quotation marks because it is actually the only medication that is specifically *not* prescribed by a physician. Rather, it is officially recommended. If a physician in any state were to actually "prescribe" for medical cannabis, he or she would be breaking the law, even in states where medical cannabis is legal.

Federal law enforced by the Food and Drug Administration (FDA) under the Controlled Substances Act (CSA) has determined cannabis to be a Schedule I narcotic with no current medical use and a high risk for addiction. Prescribing any of the Schedule I drugs, including cannabis, is currently against federal law.

> **Medical cannabis cannot legally be prescribed by a physician even in states that have legalized it. Rather, it can be officially recommended.**

STATES THAT HAVE LEGALIZED MEDICAL CANNABIS AND FEDERAL LAW

Medical cannabis has been legalized in 23 states and the District of Columbia (*see* Appendix A). However, it is still illegal under federal law, with one exception—cannabiodiol (CBD), as an extract from industrial grade hemp, can be marketed as a dietary supplement under federal and many state laws. It does not typically induce the psychoactive "high" associated with cannabis strains that are high in THC.

Currently, there are new laws being enacted in most states that will allow the use of the very low-THC, high-CBD strain of cannabis used to produce Charlotte's Web. This strain, or cultivar—as distinct from all other forms of medical marijuana, which have higher levels of THC—has very limited clinical applications and strict requirements in states where it is legal. Its use is usually restricted to the treatment of rare pediatric seizure disorders. It is unlikely for primary care clinicians to be involved in the treatment of these conditions, however.

Changing Ways to Use Medical Cannabis

Traditionally, for medical or recreational purposes, the "flowers" (buds) from the female cannabis plant have been dried and smoked. In past decades, most of the research on efficacy and safety was done using smoked flower buds. Until recently, the

FDA Schedule I status of cannabis has made research in the United States very scarce. In addition, the National Institute on Drug Abuse (NIDA) requires that the federal cannabis farm at the University of Mississippi provide the research drug. This is a significant limitation.

It is now estimated that only 40 percent of patients who use cannabis medicinally smoke it, while the other 60 percent vaporize it in a device similar to an e-cigarette; eat it as a cookie, chocolate, or sucker; or take droplets of a tincture. The smoking-related side-effects and the tell-tale aroma and social stigma are usually absent when these alternate forms are used. This trend toward the use of non-smoked medical cannabis has been a huge game-changer for patient acceptance of cannabis.

Clinical Indications for Recommending Medical Cannabis

It is recognized that cannabis can play an important role as an adjunct therapy in the treatment of chronic neuropathic or myopathic pain, anxiety, insomnia, post-traumatic stress disorder (PTSD), muscle spasms, epilepsy, multiple sclerosis (MS), inflammatory bowel disease (IBD), chemotherapy-related nausea/vomiting, AIDS, wasting syndromes, and an expanding list of cancers.

Pain is the most frequent indication. Often cannabis is not only as effective as other pain medications that are available, but it is also safer and cheaper and has fewer side-effects. In addition, cannabis has shown great promise for long-term pain control when transitioning patients off addictive and dangerous opioids.

Changing Role of Clinicians

The rapidly expanding scientific data regarding the beneficial, therapeutic effects of cannabis and its use for a widening variety of medical conditions, are making the clinician a more important player than before. Also, the increased need for monitoring and modification of treatment plans now makes it requisite for the clinician to become more involved than in the past.

The dispensary staff will eventually be relegated to dealing solely with issues of quality of product (horticultural supplies) and general patient education on the use of medical cannabis. The clinician recommending cannabinoids should have a working knowledge of the routes of delivery and therapeutic benefits of the various routes of delivery (e.g., inhalation, ingestion, oromucosal, and transdermal application). In all states where medical cannabis is legal, the clinician is the start of the process by writing a recommendation letter for a patient's use of it. Only some states allow mid-level providers to write recommendation letters. Most physicians (especially older ones) and those less exposed to patients who use cannabis, will feel uncomfortable recommending marijuana. This is especially true among physicians without specific education and experience.

> *The clinician is the start of the process in a patient's use of medical cannabis when they sign a recommendation letter, but they need to be more involved in patient follow-up.*

This text is directed toward all clinicians, but especially medical students and open-minded clinicians who are entering a new era in which patients in most, if not all, states will expect their doctors to be up to date and cooperative in recommending medical cannabis if it is clinically appropriate.

This book clarifies the history, utility, and efficacy of medical cannabis and the burgeoning new horizons for its use as a legitimate, effective, and safe medication. The reader will learn about the basic science of cannabinoids, the rapidly changing understanding of the powerful ECS, the routes for delivering cannabinoids, the pharmacology, the use of pharmacogenetic testing to select patients, and appropriate monitoring of the medication. The book's focus is on the new research and indications for use of cannabinoids in the armamentarium of practicing physicians, not on the political, social, and moral issues surrounding cannabis use.

PART I

Background and Fundamentals

CHAPTER 1

History of Human Use of Cannabis

O ver the course of human evolution many plants have been discovered to have psychoactive or medicinal effects. The earliest medications in our ancestors' pharmacopoeia were extracts from plants, including opium (codeine), foxglove (digitalis), willow bark (aspirin), and cinchona (quinine). Cannabis, with its often pungent aroma and rapid onset of effects, was bound to be discovered by our ancient ancestors.

The plant *Cannabis sativa L.* grows naturally in many tropical areas of the world, but originated in the Himalayas. Cannabis has been used for its fiber and oil-bearing seeds for 10,000 years. Cannabis plants were made into fiber for cloth and rope, and the oil from the seeds was used for a variety of household uses.

The first recorded medical use of cannabis was described in Indochinese medical texts more than 3,000 years ago. At that time it was found to be useful for a variety of both physical and mental conditions. A Chinese pharmacopoeia of the time prescribed cannabis leaves for tapeworm. Also, the seeds were pulverized and added to wine to help alleviate constipation and hair loss.

Cannabis use for recreational and medicinal effects spread throughout the Greek and Roman empires, and subsequently throughout the Islamic empire. In 440 BCE, Herodotus discussed the Scythians' use of cannabis to make a vapor for steam baths. By the Middle Ages it was regularly used externally as a balm for muscle and joint pain.

Cannabis was introduced to the Americas by the Spaniards in 1545 for use as fiber. Hemp became the first major fiber-producing plant in the United States. By 1619, King James I ordered every colonist to grow 100 plants, specifically for export. Hemp was a major crop throughout the Americas by the 18th century.

Although cannabis plants were ubiquitous throughout the United States, cannabis as a medicine did not make its way into Western medicine until 1839. At that time, Dr. William B. O'Shaughnessy returned from India with considerable experience in using cannabis for medicinal purposes. He encouraged physicians to recommend it for insomnia, pain, muscle spasms, and other physical conditions. It soon became an accepted treatment.

After its introduction and widespread acceptance into the pharmacopoeia of the time, our ancestors started to use it for a wide variety of ailments, including gonorrhea, cholera, whooping cough, and asthma. It was predominantly used as an orally ingested tincture. It is said that Queen Victoria used cannabis tincture for menstrual cramps.

The potency, efficacy, and side-effects of various medicinal preparations of cannabis extract varied significantly. For decades these tinctures were sold as "patent medicines" and therefore the ingredients were secret.

Figure 1-1 *Cannabis Indica* **Tincture**

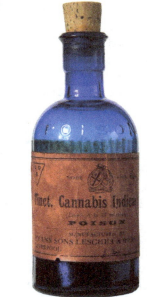

Laws Passed in the 19th and Early 20th Centuries

By the late 19th century, laws were already being enacted to address issues with purported mislabeling, adulteration, and sale of "poisons." At this time in history, smoking cannabis for recreational use in upscale hashish parlors also flourished along with opium dens.

By the beginning of the 20th century, laws in several states required prescriptions for cannabis extracts. By this time there were over 2,000 cannabis-containing preparations produced by over 280 manufacturers.

The Pure Food and Drug Act of 1906 and several state laws were passed to restrict "habit-forming drugs." This was the genesis of a series of laws to control and regulate drugs. By 1938 the Federal Pure Food, Drug, and Cosmetics Act established the framework that we still use today to regulate prescription and non-prescription drugs.

During the same period, the Marihuana Tax Act of 1937 imposed a levy of $1 per ounce on cannabis for medical use and $100 per ounce for recreational use. This law effectively made non-medical or nonindustrial use, possession, or sale of cannabis illegal throughout the United States. At that time the fledgling American Medical Association (AMA) was against this law, believing (correctly) that it would impede future medical cannabis. By 1951 the Boggs Act added cannabis to the list of narcotic drugs.

The use of marijuana for medical purposes dramatically decreased over the course of the early 20th century. There was some research in the 1950s and 1960s into its possible use for glaucoma, but far-superior ophthalmic medications became available. In the 1970s a synthetic version of tetrahydrocannabinol (THC) called *Marinol* was approved for chemotherapy-induced nausea and vomiting and later for cancer and AIDS-related cachexia. The intense psychoactive side-effects of pure THC and the patient's need to swallow oral capsules made *Marinol* a poor clinical choice, and the advent of far superior 5-HT3 and NK-1 antagonist medications made synthetic THC pharmaceuticals obsolete.

Late 20th Century Laws

In 1969, during a very turbulent period of "anti-war" social unrest, President Nixon pushed for a comprehensive restructuring of drug laws, for what he called "a war on drugs." He was especially focused on marijuana because of its association with the anti-war movement during the Vietnam era. The Controlled Substances Act (CSA) was passed into law as part of the Comprehensive Drug Abuse Prevention and Control Act of 1970. This made the possession or distribution of cannabis criminal at a federal level. This law created the five schedules of dangerous drugs (I, II, III, IV, V). The Drug Enforcement Administration (DEA) and Food and Drug Administration (FDA), together, were tasked with determining which drugs were to be included in each of the schedules. It placed cannabis in Schedule I on the grounds that the drug was deemed to have no medical use and a high risk for addiction.

When passed, this 1970 legislation effectively put an end to all serious scientific study of cannabis and severely limited the study of cannabinoids and the endocannabinoid system (ECS) when it was discovered in the early 1990s.

After several failed attempts, in 1996 California was the first state to pass legislation allowing the medicinal use of marijuana — Proposition 215, known as the Compassionate Care Act. This, along with the state's Senate Bill 420, passed in 2003, allowed for a network of growers, caregivers, health care providers, and an identification card system for use of medical marijuana in California.

Current Medical Marijuana Laws

As of the time of this writing, 23 states and the District of Columbia have some sort of legalized medical cannabis laws (*see* Appendix A). Other states allow for use of only very low-level-THC marijuana such as Charlotte's Web. The regulations and requirements vary considerably among the states, with New York allowing use of medical marijuana only if it isn't smoked. As yet, there is little scientific evidence to support the structure of the caregiver networks and most of the allowed "debilitating diseases."

There is very little human-based clinical research available to support the legislation and rules. What little recent research is available, was done using proprietary formulations of synthetic cannabinoids, not cannabis plants. That being said, the generally recognized efficacy of THC and cannabidiol (CBD) and the innate safety of these drugs has underpinned the continued support and expansion of medical marijuana laws in the United States and around the world.

In 2009, based on the rapidly evolving changes at the state level in legalization of medical cannabis, the U.S. Attorney General stated, "It will not be a priority to use federal resources to prosecute patients with serious illnesses or their caregivers who are complying with state laws on medical marijuana, but we will not tolerate drug traffickers who hide behind claims of compliance with state law to mask activities that are clearly illegal."

In December 2014, Congress and the Obama administration quietly put an end to the federal prohibition of medical cannabis use as a tiny part of a federal spending bill. However, federal banking laws still force medical dispensaries to operate as "cash only" businesses.

Most recently, the prescription-opioid epidemic ravaging the U.S. population has helped push cannabis into the spotlight as a much safer and less toxic alternative to opioids for pain control. Cannabis has been shown to be very helpful in transitioning patients off opioids.

The FDA continues to list marijuana as a Schedule I drug, but there are major efforts under way to make marijuana a Schedule II drug in the near future.

CHAPTER 2

Overview of Medical Cannabis

This chapter is a summary of the salient information about medical cannabis for clinicians. As such, it is intended to concisely introduce the clinician to the fundamentals underlying the use of cannabis as medicine. It is expected that this summary will make the reader eager to learn more about the research, concepts, issues, and subtleties of cannabis as medicine.

Cannabis, the Plant

Although the term *marijuana* is commonly used in the United States to refer to the cannabis plant, the word is actually slang. It is thought to derive from the Spanish pronunciation of the names Mary (Maria) and Jane (Juana).

PHYSICAL CHARACTERISTICS OF CANNABIS PLANTS

Cannabis has a wide variety of colors on the crystals located on the buds, the dried flower of the female plant. These colorful crystals are known as *trichomes*. Cannabis also has pungent aromas, and sometimes fruity flavors. Commonly, the aroma is an ammonia-like or skunky scent.

Cannabis sativa L. originated in the Himalayas. It is a genus of flowering herb that includes three different subspecies. However, only two subspecies, *Cannabis sativa* and *Cannabis indica*, are medically active. These two subspecies differ in their physical characteristics. *Sativa* is tall and thin and *indica* is short and bushy. The *sativa* subspecies is generally considered to be high in THC content, and *indica* high in CBD. However, with all of

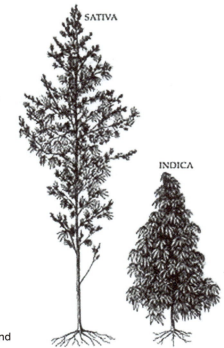

FIGURE 2-1
Comparing *Sativa* and *Indica* plants

the genetic engineering over the decades, this no longer holds true. There are innumerable hybrid strains, or cultivars, bred for different effects. The flowers (buds) and leaves have the highest concentration of cannabinoids. Very low-THC strains of cannabis have traditionally been called *hemp*. Hemp is usually a *sativa* cultivar. It has historically been used for its strong fiber, ideal for making rope and clothing, as well as for its seed oil. Since THC is the psychoactive component leading to people feeling "high," the low-THC cultivars—especially the ultra-low THC and high CBD, Charlotte's Web cultivar—are now being legalized in many states across the country for their high levels of medically active CBD.

CULTIVARS (STRAINS) OF CANNABIS

Different cultivars and even different crops of the same cultivar may have varying amounts of cannabinoids, the active components in cannabis. This means that clinical studies that use the whole plant may find different effects, depending on the cultivar used. New easy-to-use test equipment that produces quick results, such as My Dx (www.cdxlife.com/), has recently been made available for dispensaries, caregivers, and patients to quickly determine the percents of THC and CBD in the plant material. This equipment is expensive at the moment, but with time on the market and decreasing costs, it is expected to become more popular and available.

One researcher identified a wide range of ratios between THC and CBD in cannabis that was seized by law enforcement agents in California. Cannabis seized more recently had much more THC and much less CBD, compared to past seizures. This is consistent with the fact that most of this cannabis is probably currently sold and bought on the open market for recreational use.

Since the 1970s the two species have been extensively cross bred into a variety of cultivars with a broad array of interesting drug-related names. Different cultivars are often associated with different properties, at least anecdotally.

Intense breeding and genetic manipulation of cannabis cultivars has resulted in cannabis flowers (buds) that have increasingly higher content of THC. The U.S. government has said that the potency has risen 10 to 25 times, although there continues to be controversy about the average potency of cannabis bought and sold since the 1960s.

THC AND CBD POTENCY OF CANNABIS

Potency is determined by the percent of the plant material that is THC. Although the plant has a substantial amount of oil in it, most of it is comprised of dozens of cannabinoids and terpenes. Since the THC is the main psychoactive agent associated with many medicinal effects as well as the most potent side-effects, the potency of a cultivar usually depends on the THC level. In addition, because CBD also has medicinal effects and modifies THC effects, the percentage of CBD is also important. Usually, the CBD and THC percentages in the bud will be specified by the cannabis dispensary, along with the number of milligrams of the product (plant oil, tincture, or edible).

The University of Mississippi has an ongoing Potency Monitoring Project. In 2009 cannabis seized from all 50 states was tested to determine potency. The average potency was 8.52 percent THC in 2009 and 1.37 percent in 1978. A review over the years at the Potency Monitoring Project has shown that some newer cultivars grown under special circumstances may have as high as 37.2 percent potency. However, with the increasing potency of the plant material, the amount of cannabis smoked or vaporized by people who use it has declined. People tend to naturally titrate the dose by the psychoactive effects, using a series of closely spaced inhalations (hits) of a pipe, vaporizer, or cannabis cigarette.

If the patient is going to use plant material by either smoking or vaporizing it, he or she should be given basic advice on how to calculate the recommended THC or CBD dose that will be obtained from different cannabis cultivars. The dispensary will almost always provide information on the percent potency of the cannabis flowers that are being dispensed. However, these percentages of THC and CBD may be inaccurate, as there are still no generally applied standards for testing of potency.

There are almost 500 identifiable chemical constituents known to exist in cannabis plants. Around 85 of these are phyto-cannabinoids, or cannabinoids of plant origin. The cannabinoid CBD can make up to 30 percent of the plant's extractable material. Other than THC and CBD, the dozens of other cannabinoids are present in only small amounts. The majority of these compounds have not been well studied.

AROMATIC TERPENES

Aromatic terpenes are also present in the plant material. Over 120 different terpenes have been identified in cannabis. They comprise 10 to 29 percent of the oils produced by the plant. It is these aromatic terpenes that drug-sniffing dogs have been trained to detect. Several of the terpenes in cannabis are known to have medicinal effects. These terpenes are also found in a wide variety of other plants (fruits, flowers, and spices). The most prevalent terpene is Myrcene, which has a mango scent. Other prevalent terpenes are Borneol, which has a camphor scent, and Eucalyptol, with a minty smell. Caryophyllene smells like black pepper and has been shown to bind with CB2 receptors, similar to CBD. It has recently been approved as a food additive by the FDA and is in clinical trials for reducing neuropathic pain.

There are many other aromatic terpenes. In general these terpenes, other than Caryophyllene, are not believed to contribute significantly to the pharmaceutical effects of cannabis. However, ongoing research suggests that they may assist in the efficacy of the medical cannabinoids, via the entourage effect.

Other plants besides cannabis are known to have cannabinoids. However, these are not the medically active THC or CBD cannabinoids.

The Endocannabinoid System (ECS)

A little more than 20 years ago, researchers discovered a natural system in the brain and body that has receptors for the active components of cannabis. They named it the *endocannabinoid system (ECS)*. The ECS is involved with several important and sometimes unique aspects of physiology, immunology, psychology, and even tumor suppression. The physiologic processes that are germane for clinicians are appetite, pain sensation, mood, memory, gastrointestinal functions, inflammatory response, and immune function.

The existence of the ECS is the bedrock rationale underlying the medicinal use of cannabis. Therefore, a separate chapter (Chapter 3) is devoted to it. In this overview, it is sufficient to explain that the ECS receptors, CB1 and CB2, respond in medically beneficial ways to endocannabinoids naturally produced by the body, phytocannabinoids from the cannabis plants, and the newer synthetic cannabinoids developed by pharmaceutical companies. The two most extensively studied phytocannabinoids are THC and CBD. THC stimulates CB1 receptors in the brain and to a lesser extent in the body. CBD has little affinity for either receptor, but it indirectly increases the amount of natural endocannabinoid at the CB1 and CB2 receptors.

Phytocannabinoids in Cannabis

As previously mentioned, the plant *Cannabis sativa L.* is a genus of flowering herb that includes three different subspecies, but only two subspecies, *Cannabis sativa* and *Cannabis indica,* are medically active. Intense breeding and genetic manipulation of cannabis cultivars over the past two decades has resulted in cannabis flowers (buds) that have an increasingly higher content of THC. There are almost 500 identifiable chemical constituents known to exist in cannabis plants. Around 85 of these are phytocannabinoids.

THC is the only psychoactive agent in cannabis and is associated with many beneficial medical effects. The most potent side-effects also derive from the THC level. The CBD level is important in modifying the psychoactive effects of THC effects. Increasing the ratio of CBD to THC tends to reduce the psychoactive effects of THC. In general, combining CBD with THC results in a medication that has many fewer side-effects.

Since THC is the psychoactive component that causes users of cannabis to feel "high," growers have been developing low-THC cultivars, especially the ultra-low-THC, high-CBD cultivar known as *Charlotte's Web*. This low-THC cultivar and similar cultivars are now being legalized across the country for their high levels of medically active CBD.

Development of Cannabinoid Pharmaceuticals

By the 1980s dromabinol (Marinol) and nabilone (Cesamet), both synthetic THC analogues, had been patented by pharmaceutical companies for treatment of chemotherapy-related nausea and vomiting (CINV), and they were later approved for stimulation of appetite. Many other THC analogues were developed, but because they had significant psychoactive effects they were deemed unsuitable for pharmaceutical purposes.

The naturally-occurring combinations of THC, CBD, and terpenes in the cannabis plant is believed to be far superior to these man-made pharmaceuticals.

Burgeoning Developments in Pharmacogenetics

Pharmacogenetics is the study of individual variations in the genetic sequence as they relate to drug response. Pharmacogenetic testing involves identification of various alternative and mutant forms of alleles of genes and the enzymes in them that are involved in the metabolism of medications. This is a keystone in the rapidly evolving area of personalized medicine. There are several enzymes in the cytochrome P450 system and certain CB1 variants associated with increased risk of cannabis dependence and its associated psychosis, as well as drug-drug interactions with THC and CBD. Although the field of pharmacogenetics is still in its infancy, it may become a regular part of the clinical practice of cannabis medication management.

Research on the Use of Cannabis as Medicine

There are very few high-quality studies to support the use of medical cannabis for the variety of conditions for which it has been recommended. Most of the studies that have been performed have predominately used animal models, with small numbers of patients, and were done decades ago with poor methodology or using synthetic pharmaceutical cannabinoids, not plant material. The more recent studies are also largely animal-based *in vivo* or *in vitro* studies, but plant-based cannabinoids are finally the source of very intense study, and new clinical studies are forthcoming.

For a detailed summary of the basic science and clinical research on cannabis as medicine, Health Canada published *Information for Health Care Professionals* in 2013 (www.hc-sc.gc .ca/dhp-mps/marihuana/med/infoprof-eng.php#chp221).

Role of Medical Cannabis in Clinical Practice

USE AS ADJUNCT THERAPY

Currently, medical cannabis should never be used as first-line treatment for any condition. Rather, it plays a supportive role, along with other more generally recognized therapies, for treatment of specific symptoms or medical conditions.

Both THC and CBD are very safe when used appropriately, with relatively mild short-term side-effects from an excessive dose or accidental ingestion. When recommending cannabis therapy, the clinician needs to be cognizant of the possible development of cannabis dependency syndrome and associated psychosis. The main side-effect of THC lies in its psychoactive properties, resulting in the person using it to feel "high." In general, this side-effect tends to lessen over time and with experience in titrating the medicine. The only documented side-effect of CBD is sedation at high doses and the potential for immunosuppression; the latter has been unconfirmed by high-quality research studies, however.

Both THC and CBD are non-lethal, regardless of the route of administration when ingested. This is because, unlike opioids and benzodiazepines, there are no endocannabinoid receptors in the brain stem, so there is no depressant respiratory effect.

> *Since cannabis is a Schedule I Controlled Substance at the federal level, it is against DEA and FDA regulations to "prescribe it," even if it is legal under state law to use it for medical purposes. The clinician only recommends cannabis in a standard format letter (see Appendix B).*

Medical cannabis is much less expensive than recreational cannabis—generally about half the price. Many patients requesting cannabis for medical conditions are probably doing so to obtain it primarily for their own recreational purposes or to sell to others. Physicians need to guard against the possibilities of this fact and act accordingly.

If and when Sativex is FDA approved, it will be the first prescription cannabis medication with effects similar to cannabis products available at cannabis dispensaries. However, it will be available at community pharmacies and will likely be covered for several conditions by health insurance.

ROUTES OF ADMINISTRATION, DOSING, AND SIDE-EFFECTS

These are discussed in detail in Chapters 6, 9, and 13.

CHAPTER 3

The Endocannabinoid System

One of the most exciting new developments in the field of cannabis as medicine has been the discovery of the endocannabinoid system (ECS). In 1990 the first endogenous THC-sensitive receptor was discovered in rats. In the past two decades there has been an exponential increase in our understanding of how the ECS works and its role in several important and sometimes unique areas of physiology, immunology, psychology, and even tumor suppression. The ECS is involved with a variety of physiologic processes, including appetite, pain sensation, mood, memory, gastrointestinal functions, inflammatory response, and immune function.

Unfortunately, most of the research has been in *in vivo* animal or *in vitro* tissue culture. Since the 1970s almost all NIH supported research related to cannabis were designed to prove the deleterious effects of cannabis, while blocking research into the beneficial effects. It is estimated that only 8 percent of the older studies focused on the therapeutic benefits of cannabis, although this has changed considerably in recent years.

What is the ECS?

The ECS is like several other neuromodulatory systems in the body, such as the adrenergic and dopaminergic systems. The ECS has ligands, receptors, and enzymatic degradation of the ligands. We now know that the ECS is comprised of at least three neuromodulators and at least two receptors, CB1 and CB2 (and possibly four). The receptors are found predominantly in the brain but also, to some extent, throughout the body, especially in the immune system. The neuromodulators are anandamide

(AEA), 2-arachidonoylglycerol (2-AG), and palmitoylethanol-amide (PEA).

AEA is the principal ligand for CB1, whose effects, which are primarily in the central nervous system (CNS), are discussed below. 2-AG is the principal ligand of CB2, primarily in the immune-system cell lines. Palmitoylethanolamide is not strictly an endocannabinoid. It has an affinity for G protein-coupled receptor 55 (GPR55), which may soon be called *CB3*. However, it lacks affinity for CB1 or CB2. Its presence has been shown to enhance the effects of AEA by the so-called entourage effect. Its effects are primarily anti-inflammatory and anti-nociceptive, primarily through reduction of mast cells' infiltration and activation and inhibition of dorsal root ganglia activation.

Plant-based cannabinoids, also called *phytocannabinoids*—primarily delta-9-tetrahydrocannabinol (THC), cannabidiol (CBD), and cannabinol (CBN)—are discussed in Chapter 4.

The Entourage Effect

The *entourage effect* refers to the observation of the synergistic or modulating effects that occur when several of the related cannabinoids are present at one time, as opposed to the effects when just one isolated cannabinoid is present at the receptors. The research suggests that they work together at a chemical and cellular level. For example, the concomitant presence of CBD with THC in naturally occurring cannabis (the plant) tends to decrease the psychoactive effects of the THC by means of the entourage effect.

With cannabis, not only are the dozens of cannabinoids important, but studies have shown that the plethora of terpenoids present in the cannabis plant also contribute to the entourage effect.

The cannabinoid receptors are present on the pre-synaptic membranes. The higher the level of expression of cannabinoid receptors, the more efficient the ligand coupling, and thus the more potent the effects of the cannabinoids.

Unlike most hormonal feedback systems, the ECS is a retrograde system that, when stimulated, produces an inhibitory effect on neurotransmitters, which dampens or decreases the excitatory effect of the neurotransmitters. The other neurotransmitters, however, may be inhibitory or excitatory.

In the ECS the post-synaptic neuron releases the endocannabinoids in retrograde transmission, which binds them to the pre-synaptic cannabinoid receptors. This reduces the amount of the other neurotransmitter that is released and thus its associated neuronal excitability. For example, stimulation of the CB2 receptors results in the inhibition of the immune response and inflammation cascades. It is believed that the ECS plays a vital role in modulating neurotransmitter release to maintain homeostasis and in preventing excessive neuronal activity.

There is good evidence that the ECS receptors can inhibit ongoing release of a number of different excitatory and inhibitory neurotransmitters, including acetylcholine, dopamine, noradrenaline, gaba-aminobutyric acid (GABA), and 5-hydroxytryptamine (5-HT).

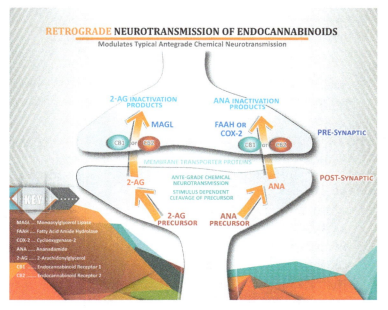

Figure 3-1 Retrograde Neurotransmission of Endocannabinoids

THC and CBD:
The Most Studied Cannabinoids

The CB1 and CB2 receptors respond to the endocannabinoids naturally produced by the body (endogenous cannabinoids), to phytocannabinoids from the cannabis plant, and to the newer synthetic cannabinoids developed by pharmaceutical companies. The two most extensively studied phytocannabinoids are THC and CBD, although there is also an increasing interest in CBN. THC stimulates CB1 receptors in the brain and, to a lesser extent, in the body. CBD has little affinity for either receptor, but it suppresses AEA hydrolysis by fatty acid amide hydrolase (FAAH), thereby increasing the amount of endocannabinoid at the CB1 receptors. CBD also stimulates the release of 2-AG that activates both CB1 and CB2 receptors. In addition, CBD has high affinity for GPR55.

Although CBD does not bind to the known cannabinoid receptors, it directly interacts with other G-protein-coupled receptors. Specifically, it binds to the TRPV-1 receptor, which mediates neuropathic pain perception, inflammation, and body temperature. TRPV-1, known as the *capsaicin receptor*, is the same neuropathic pain modulator that capsaicin activates.

CBN has not been as well studied as THC and CBD. It is weakly psychoactive and is found only in trace amounts in cannabis. It is a metabolite of THC. CBN acts as a weak agonist of CB1 receptors but has a higher affinity for CB2 receptors, with lower affinity compared to THC.

CB1 Receptors

Cannabinoid receptor 1 (CB1) is present in varying degrees in several structures within the brain. The following is a fairly complete list of these:

- Amygdala: regulates anxiety and fear.
- Basal ganglia: regulates reaction time.
- Brain stem: regulates nausea effects.
- Cerebellum: regulates coordination and balance.
- Hippocampus: regulates short-term memory.
- Hypothalamus: involved in appetite and sexual behavior.
- Neocortex: involved in complex thinking and judgment.

- Nucleus accumbens: regulates reward and pleasure sensation.
- Spinal cord: regulates pain perception.

CB1 receptors are also present in peripheral organs but to a much lesser extent. They are present in peripheral neurons. They are found in the uterus, pancreas, liver, gastrointestinal (GI) tract, and adipose tissue. CB1 regulates psychoactive, central nervous system (CNS), and some anticonvulsive effects.

CB2 Receptors

CB2 receptors are found on leukocytes and throughout the body in the immune-system cell lines, especially B cells, natural killer cells, and mast cells. CB2 receptors are also found in the spleen and peripheral nervous system and are present, to some extent, throughout the visceral organ systems and GI tract. They are also present to a limited extent in the CNS.

In the immune system, the ECS modulates cytokine production, immune cell migration, and apoptosis, a form of tightly regulated cell suicide. In mast cells, CB2 receptors modulate the inflammatory response. In the GI tract, activation of the CB2 receptors results in reduction of noradrenaline release, concomitant regulation of intestinal motility, and smooth muscle contractions in the urinary and reproductive systems.

GPR55 Receptors

Recent research suggests that an additional binding receptor, G protein-coupled receptor 55 (GPR55), is widely present in the brain, especially the cerebellum. In the periphery, its expression appears to be limited to the small intestine as well as osteoclasts and osteoblasts in the bone marrow. It has been shown to be involved with bone cell regulation. However, most of its physiologic effects are unknown.

GPR55 may soon be categorized as the CB3 receptor. It is activated by the naturally occurring endocannabinoids AEA and 2-AG and by the phytocannabinoids THC and CBD.

AEA

AEA is the principal ligand of CB1 receptors, especially in the brain. In the periphery it is also a CB2 ligand. It is widely present in the CNS, including the hippocampus, where it is involved with short-term memory; the hypothalamus, where it is involved with the pleasure associated with food; the limbic system, where it is involved with responses to stressors; the nucleus accumbens, where it is involved with reward associated with food; the basal ganglia, where it is involved with sleep onset; and the cortex, where it has many functions related to nociception and response to stressors. Elevated levels of AEA are believed to have a beneficial effect on both anxiety and depression.

In the periphery it has been found in several organ systems. AEA has an important function related to implantation of an early-stage embryo in the uterus. It has also been identified in the cardiovascular system, in the GI tract, and in adipose tissue. Although much of this research is in its infancy, AEA is present in very low levels in the body because of its rapid breakdown. It is degraded by FAAH. Therefore, inhibitors of FAAH lead to increased levels of AEA and CB1 activation. Dietary AEA found in chocolate and other food items causes increased AEA levels in the body. High-fat diets have also been associated with elevated levels, and elevated levels have been associated with the development of obesity.

Acetaminophen is metabolically combined with arachidonic acid by FAAH. Acetaminophen is a potent agonist of transient receptor potential cation channel, subfamily V, member 1 (TRPV-1), which is involved with neuropathic pain, and is an inhibitor of AEA re-uptake. These actions are felt to be partially or fully responsible for the analgesic effects of acetaminophen.

2-AG

2-AG is present in high levels in the brain but is also found in the periphery. It is a full agonist of CB1 and CB2 receptors. It is the primary ligand for CB2 receptors in the periphery. It plays an important role in modulating neuropathic pain in the spinal cord. It also has several modulating effects on immune system cells. 2-AG is very important in the inflammatory response of mast cells and in the intestinal tract. Elevated levels of 2-AG found in patients with closed head injury were associated with a neuroprotective effect and improved outcomes.

2-AG is hydrolyzed mostly by monoacyglycerol lipase (MAGL), and, to a much lesser extent, by FAAH.

Palmitoylethanolamide (PEA)

Because PEA lacks affinity for CB1 and CB2, it is not considered a classic endocannabinoid. However, it has a variety of clinically positive functions related to nociception and inflammation via GPR55 (CB3?). PEA was discovered decades before the ECS. In the 1970s several efforts were made to produce a PEA-based pharmaceutical for pain and inflammation, and also for influenza prophylaxis. It appears to work synergistically with AEA in its nociceptive effects.

Transient Receptor Potential Vanilloid Receptor 1 (TRPV-1)

TRPV-1 is also known as the *capsaicin receptor*. It is involved with neuropathic pain perception and thermoregulation of the body. Activation of TRPV-1 receptors leads to painful, burning sensations. TRPV-1 receptors are found in the CNS and the peripheral nervous system. AEA and cannabis-based CBD have been shown to directly or indirectly activate TRPV-1 receptors. This is discussed in more detail in Chapter 8 on pain.

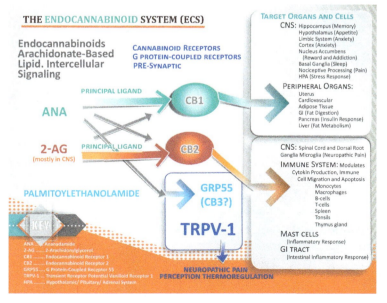

Figure 3-2 The Endocannabinoid System (ECS)

Research has shown that the ECS is involved with the physiology and function of many organs and systems.

The current research suggests that hypothalamic neurons continually produce endocannabinoids that work to regulate hunger. Other studies have shown that the amount of endocannabinoids produced is inversely correlated with the amount of leptin in the blood and thus is associated with hedonic pleasure of sweet taste in the nucleus accumbens. Taken together the research shows that cannabinoid activity in the brain is strongly related to food-seeking behavior.

New basic research has shown that endocannabinoids help the hypopituitary-adrenal axis habituate to stress, reducing the corticosteroid response to repeated or nonthreatening stressors.

The ECS has been shown to have anxiolytic effects by inhibiting excessive arousal in response to novel situations. Other research has shown that CBD activates adenosine receptors in the brain, down-regulating the release of anxiety-related neurotransmitters, dopamine, and glutamate. At high concentrations, CBD directly triggers an inhibitory response on 5-HT1A serotonin signaling. This results in beneficial effects on depression.

Another area of research is immune function. Endocannabinoids have been shown to have immunomodulator effects on the immune system. The ECS is involved with pain perception. At the spinal cord, cannabinoids suppress noxious-stimulus-evoked responses of neurons in the dorsal horn, possibly by modulating descending noradrenaline input from the brain stem.

The discovery of the ECS has produced strong motivation among scientists to conduct basic and clinical research into the use of cannabinoids for medical purposes.

Endocannabinoid Deficiency

Although much basic and clinical research still needs to be done, University of Washington neurologist Ethan Russo has postulated that "clinical endocannabinoid deficiency" is a real condition, which could underlie irritable bowel syndrome, a variety of degenerative conditions, migraine headaches, and fibromyalgia.

Much more basic science and clinical research needs to be conducted. But there is great promise in the further study of THC and CBD and eventually other phytocannabinoids.

Question about How Medical Cannabis Works

Dr. Wong is standing in line with you in the hospital cafeteria. He says he is uncomfortable recommending cannabis in his primary care practice. He knows that you regularly use it in carefully selected and managed patients. He wants to know how medical cannabis works. What can you tell him in 30 seconds?

Discussion: Thirty seconds is just enough time to tell Dr. Wong that there is an endogenous system for naturally occurring cannabinoids called the *endocannabinoid system* (ECS). Unlike most feedback systems in the body, the ECS is a retrograde feedback system that, when stimulated, produces an inhibitory effect on other neurotransmitters. This reduces the amount of neurotransmitter released and associated neuronal excitability. So far we know of at least two ECS receptors, CB1 and CB2. THC and CBD are the two most studied cannabinoids in cannabis. There are many other cannabinoids in cannabis; they act much like plant-based hormones on hormone receptors. In general, THC stimulates CB1 receptors in the brain, and CBD stimulates CB2 receptors in the body's other organ systems. However, it is much more complex than this.

Because of historical legal and DEA drug scheduling issues, there is a dearth of good studies on cannabis. However, the body of evidence suggests that it may be beneficial and sometimes very effective for an expanding array of medical conditions and symptoms.

CHAPTER 4

Plant-Based Cannabinoids

Cannabis plants produce large amounts of phytocannabi-noids, or plant-based cannabinoids. The cannabinoids are present mostly in the viscous resin produced in the plant's glandular structures, the trichomes. These are the colorful crystalline structures that give the pungent aroma and often vivid variety of colors to the cannabis buds.

THC and CBD

These chemicals, predominantly THC and CBD, are the medically active components of the plant material. As much as 30 percent of the resin is CBD. In addition, if cannabis is ingested, at least 50 percent of the THC will be metabolized in the liver to 11-hydroxy-delta-9-tetrahydrocannabinol (11-OH-THC), which has a much stronger affinity for some cannabinoid receptors than THC. It is considered the main active ingredient when cannabis is orally ingested. When THC is exposed to the air for long periods of time, it oxidizes to cannabinol (CBN), which has only very weak psychoactive effects and is, otherwise, much like CBD.

Mechanisms of Action and Properties

The phytocannabinoids act very much like the naturally occur-ring endocannabinoids, AEA and 2-AG. However, phytocan-nabinoids target cannabinoid receptors in a far less selective manner than the endocannabinoids. In addition, the pharma-cologic effect of phytocannabinoids is dependent on the density and the coupling efficiency of the cannabinoid receptors in the organ or brain center. The available evidence shows that the density or coupling efficiency varies significantly in different centers of the brain.

Because THC is only a partial agonist, it may have antagonistic effects on the endogenous ligands (AEA and 2-A6) in areas of the brain.

The main psychoactive cannabinoid is THC, which includes both delta-9-tetrahydrocannabinol and delta-8-tetrahydrocannabinol. It mimics the effects of AEA, binding to CB1 receptors in the brain, and modulates CB2 receptors in the body with about equal affinity. Research suggests that it has moderate analgesic effects, stimulates the appetite, and has marked antiemetic properties.

The fact that THC is only a partial agonist may result in antagonistic effects on the endogenous ligands (AEA and 2-AG) in areas of the brain where there is low expression of receptors, or poor coupling efficiency. Certain disorders or diseases can result in up-regulation of cannabinoid receptors and, over time, increased cannabinoid response. For example, chronic neuropathic pain is associated with increased expression of

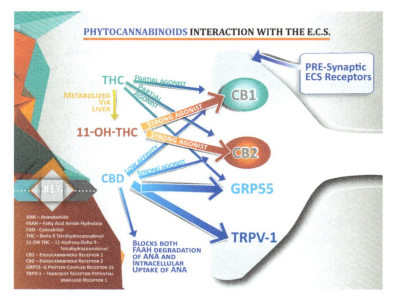

Figure 4-1 Phytocannabinoids' Interaction with the ECS

cannabinoid receptors in the thalamus, spinal cord, and dorsal root ganglia.

Repeat exposure of cannabinoid receptors to ligands (natural or plant-based) can lead to a decrease in receptor density and coupling efficiency. This can manifest as tolerance. The down-regulation of the receptors varies in different parts of the brain and organ systems. Some areas of the brain or organ systems may be less down-regulated than others, which is often beneficial pharmacologically—for example, if tolerance to the psychoactive effects of THC develop early, and tolerance to the appetite-stimulant effects take much longer.

Phytocannabinoids are a diverse class of chemical compounds that bind to the cannabinoid receptors, CB1 and CB2, in the ECS. In addition, they bind to G-protein-couple receptor 55 (GPR55). There is another cannabinoid receptor that was recently discovered in the hippocampus; it has not yet been cloned and may eventually be named *CB4*.

CBD

CBD has only low affinity for CB1 and CB2. However, CBD blocks the degradation of the endocannabinoid AEA by the enzyme fatty acid amide hydrolase (FAAH). It also blocks the intracellular uptake of AEA. The result of these two effects is an increase in the available naturally occurring AEA at the cannabinoid receptors. In addition, recent research shows that CBD has an unexpectedly high potency as a CB2-receptor antagonist. CBD has been shown to be an agonist of GPR55, which is present in the brain and peripherally on osteoblasts and osteoclasts.

As a ligand of transient receptor potential cation channel subfamily V member 1 (TRPV-1), also known as the *capsaicin receptor*, CBD also has effects outside of the ECS. It is through these effects that CBD modulates heat nociception and neuropathic pain perception. CBD's many effects on nociception and inflammation make it a prime target for a new class of anti-inflammatory agents.

Phytocannabinoids imitate some effects of endocannabinoids.

Chemically, phytocannabinoids are all aromatic terpenoids, with low-water solubility. They have excellent solubility in organic solvents. They can be total or partial ligands of the ECS receptors. They imitate some of the effects of the naturally occurring endocannabinoids anandamide (AEA), 2-arachidonoylglycerol (2-AG), and palmitoylethanolamide (PEA), depending on which receptors they bind.

How much effect THC or CBD has on an organ system, or a part of the brain, is strongly influenced by the expression level and signaling efficiency of the cannabinoid receptors and by ongoing natural endocannabinoid release.

THC and CBD work together.

The ratio of the amount of THC to CBD in the plant material has become important to understanding the effects of each of these cannabinoids. The two cannabinoids work together. For example, people using pure THC preparations such as Marinol have much more anxiety and psychoactive effects, compared to those who use a natural compound with a ratio of 1:1 THC to CBD. Increasing the ratio of CBD to THC tends to reduce the psychoactive effects of THC. In general, combining CBD with THC results in a medication that has many fewer side-effects.

The trend over the past decades has been to develop cultivars with very low-THC, such as Charlotte's Web, for medical purposes. At the same time, recreational users of cannabis have pushed for the development of cultivars very high in THC, with ratios as high as 20:1 for THC to CBD. The presence and/or ratio of the two cannabinoids cannot be determined by smell, taste, or feel. Dispensary staff will often attribute potent medical effects to brightly colored or pungent strains of cannabis. These smells and colors are usually due to the secondary terpenes, not to the medically active THC and CBD in the cannabis.

Terpenes and Other Cannabinoids

It has been postulated that the wide variety of other terpenes present in the plant material alters the properties of both CBD and THC. However, research into the optimal cannabinoid ratios and the interaction of cannabinoids with terpenes is still in its infancy.

Sativex is a new pharmaceutical readily available in Europe. It contains a 1:1 ratio of naturally occurring THC and CBD in addition to naturally occurring terpenes. Sativex has been used effectively for pain control, muscle spasms, and insomnia.

Other Cannabinoids

There are at least 85 different cannabinoids present in cannabis plants. These other phytocannabinoids are present in only minute quantities, but many have been shown to have affinity for cannabinoid receptors. In addition to THC and CBD, there are several other phytocannabinoids with which the clinician should be familiar: Some of the other cannabinoids present in cannabis include cannabigerol (CBG), cannabinol (CBN), tetrahydrocannabinolic acid (THCA), tetrahydrocannabivarin (THCV), and cannabidivarin (CBDV). These are often listed on the chemical analysis of cannabis plant material from dispensaries. There has been little hard research conducted to study these chemicals. For the most part, these other cannabinoids are not psychoactive; their effects are similar to those of CBD. Future research may provide information about the medical utility of these chemicals.

CBG

CBG, which is not psychoactive, is present in high amounts in hemp plants. It has been shown to reduce intraocular pressure and to have positive effects on inflammatory bowel disease.

CBN

CBN is found in only trace amounts in cannabis. It is a metabolite of THC. It has weak psychoactive effects. It has been shown to be a partial agonist of CB2 receptors and a weak agonist of CB1 receptors.

THCA

THCA is the precursor of THC. It is present in moderate amounts in fresh cannabis but gradually decarboxylates to THC as it dries out and under intense heat from vaporization or smoking. In a laboratory analysis of cannabis, the percentage of THC is added to the THCA percentage to determine the cannabis's potency.

THCA does not have psychoactive effects but does have anti-inflammatory, neuroprotective, and antiemetic properties.

THCV

THCV is a homologue of THC. It is found in significant amounts in fresh cannabis. Like THC, it is a CB1 and CB2 partial agonist. The psychoactive effects of THCV are not well characterized. An older study performed on rats suggests that it may be beneficial for weight loss and for reducing fasting insulin levels. Studies are currently being conducted to develop a THCV-based pharmaceutical for weight loss.

SYNTHETIC CANNABIS

The pharmacologic characterization of phytocannabinoids in the 1970s subsequently led to the development of synthetic cannabinoids. By the 1980s, dromabinol (Marinol) and nabilone (Cesamet), both THC analogues, had been patented by pharmaceutical companies for treatment of chemo-induced nausea and vomiting (CINV) and were later approved for stimulation of appetite. Many other analogues of THC were created. These had significant psychoactive effects and were deemed unsuitable for pharmaceutical purposes.

HERBAL INCENSE

In the past decade, several of these previously known psychoactive artificial, chemical cannabinoids have been used as designer drugs. The chemical is sprayed on herbs and labeled "herbal incense," then sold for recreational purposes. Since these products are incense and not to be consumed, they were initially legal to sell. The products are commonly known as synthetic cannabis. The two most common of these products, K2 and Spice, are sold throughout the country in "smoke shops" and convenience stores. Synthetic cannabinoids, such as JWH-018 and JWH-073, mimic the effects of THC via agonist effects on the ECS.

These particular synthetic cannabinoids are very dangerous, resulting in an increasing number of emergency department visits around the country. Unlike THC, they have been deadly. Studies show that many of these agents can precipitate psychosis. They are not detected in standard urine drug tests for THC.

The most common symptoms after smoking "herbal incense" are tachycardia, elevated blood pressure, nausea, blurred vision, hallucinations, and agitation. The greatly increased side-effects of these agents is due to the fact that they tend to be full agonists of the ECS, compared to THC, which is only a partial agonist and not able to saturate and activate all of the receptors. In addition, the metabolites of some of the synthetic cannabinoids may increase their toxicity, compared to THC. Persistent psychosis for weeks or months can occur after use of synthetic cannabinoids. The clinician should consider questioning patients about possible synthetic cannabinoid use in the scenario of acute-onset or persistent psychosis.

These synthetic cannabinoids are quickly being outlawed throughout the United States and in Europe. There are dozens of chemicals within various classes that can mimic THC, and new ones are constantly surfacing in attempts to by-pass the laws. In July 2012, the Synthetic Drug Abuse Prevention Act of 2012 was signed into law. It banned synthetic compounds commonly found in synthetic cannabis, placing them under Schedule I of the Controlled Substances Act.

Dravet Syndrome

A parent of a patient with Dravet syndrome is following up for a re-evaluation of his son. He tells you that he is growing his own cannabis and is not certain that it is the low-THC strain. He wants to know if it will still be effective if the strain he is growing has more than a small amount of THC in it. What can you tell him?

Discussion: Dravet is one of a number of seizure disorders for which medical cannabis has been shown to be effective. For Dravet, it may be the only drug that works, after all conventional medications have been tried.

However, it is the CBD, not the THC, that is having the anti-seizure effect. Preparations of pure CBD are available, many of them over-the-counter for use in small handheld vaporizers. Also, the cultivar Charlotte's Web is very high in CBD, with almost no intoxicating THC. He should stick to these preparations, which are known to be very low in THC.

The use of cannabis with higher levels of THC, a strain of which he may be unknowingly growing at home, can cause significant adverse psychoactive effects, dependency, and future cognitive issues in children and adolescents using it regularly.

CHAPTER 5

Cannabis Pharmaceuticals

There are currently a couple of FDA-approved cannabinoid-based pharmaceuticals that have been around for over two decades. In addition, several non-FDA-approved medications have been used successfully in Europe and are bound to make their way through the FDA approval process. It is interesting to note that even though cannabis is a Schedule I agent, these pharmaceuticals are on Schedule II and III.

Synthetic Cannabis Medications

Most primary care clinicians will not be using these specialized medications, since they are for cancer-related or HIV-related conditions. In addition, these are ancient medications in today's pharmacopeia, relatively speaking, and other far-superior non-cannabinoid medications are available for these conditions. These medications are based on synthetic cannabinoids, thus not obtained from the cannabis plant. They have significant side-effects compared to use of plant-based cannabis medication; they are very expensive; and they carry a higher risk for physical dependence than the plant-based medications.

The synthetic THC pharmaceuticals are discussed for the sake of completeness and to provide some historical perspective of our understanding of the pharmacology of cannabinoid medications.

The primary care clinician should have a basic knowledge of these medications. Unlike cannabis-derived medications, these are made from synthetic analogues of THC, and each one is patented and FDA approved. Therefore, they can be prescribed, and no recommendation letter is necessary. Also, unlike cannabis, their use is reimbursed by health insurance companies.

The two THC analogues have been shown to have worse psychoactive effects to marijuana, which limits their clinical application.

It should be recalled that the naturally occurring combinations of THC, CBD, and terpenes in plant-based medicine are far superior to these man-made pharmaceuticals, mainly due to the lack of entourage effect. The more recent studies have repeatedly shown the importance of the THC-to-CBD ratio as well as the entourage effects of the terpenes. In addition, the dozens of other cannabinoids present in small amounts in plant-based medicine probably have associated medical effects. These possible effects require further quality research.

Unfortunately, many of the studies of medical cannabinoids from the 1990s focus on proprietary synthetic single-cannabinoid drugs. Therefore, the study results are not necessarily transferable to plant-based cannabis medication.

Marinol

(www.webmd.com/drugs/2/drug-9308/marinol-oral/details)
Marinol (generic name: dronabinol) is manufactured by Unimed Pharmaceuticals. It became available in 1985. It is synthetically manufactured THC analogue. It comes in 2.5-mg, 5-mg, and 10-mg soft gelatin capsules. Sesame oil is an inactive ingredient in the preparation.

INDICATIONS
Marinol was originally FDA approved to stimulate appetite in wasting conditions such as AIDS and cancer-related anorexia. It subsequently became FDA approved to treat nausea and vomiting for chemotherapy-related side effects. It has been widely used off-label over the years for multiple sclerosis (MS)-related spasms and neuropathic pain. It is FDA approved on Schedule III.

DOSING
For stimulating appetite, the usual starting dose is 2.5 mg before lunch and before dinner. If the patient experiences unpleasant psychoactive effects, the dosing can be reduced to once-a-day dosing, 2.5 mg before dinner *or* at bedtime, because of the long

half-life of the appetite-stimulating effect. For increased effect, the dosing can be gradually adjusted to 5 mg at breakfast, then 5 mg at lunch and at dinner. The maximum dose is 40 mg a day.

Studies of AIDS patients show increased body weight, elevated mood, and decreased nausea. Sustained efficacy for the appetite-stimulating effects has been shown to last for at least five months.

For chemotherapy-induced nausea and vomiting (CINV), the usual starting dose is 5 mg per meter squared, given 1–3 hours prior to administration of chemotherapy. This is followed every 2–4 hours after chemotherapy for a total of four to six doses. If the starting dose is ineffective, following doses can be increased to 2.5 mg per meter-squared increments, up to a maximum of 15 mg per meter squared per dose. Marinol can be combined with other antiemetic medications such as prochlorperazine for additive effects, as well as to decrease side-effects from higher doses of these medications used alone.

SIDE-EFFECTS

Because it is essentially pure THC, Marinol can have side-effects, namely, increased sympathomimetic effects such as tachycardia and conjunctival injection. Orthostatic hypotension has also been reported.

In addition, patients report a dose-related "high" marked by outbursts of laughing, elation, and heightened awareness.

EFFICACY

Marinol has dose-related effects on appetite, antiemetic effects, and psychoactive effects on cognition, memory, and perception. There is great patient-to-patient variation in response to the medication. Patients usually develop tolerance to the unpleasant side-effects of Marinol within two weeks. However, tolerance to the appetite-stimulating effects does not develop very quickly.

Marinol is orally administered and has an onset of action after 30–60 minutes and peak effect at 2–4 hours. There is a large first-pass hepatic effect, and only 10 to 20 percent of the dose reaches the circulation. The psychoactive effects tend to last 4–6 hours, while the effect of appetite stimulation can last 24 hours or longer.

SPECIAL POPULATIONS

Pediatric and Geriatric Patients

Marinol has not been studied in pediatric populations. Because of issues with its psychoactive effects, caution should be observed when using Marinol in pediatric patients. There is an increasing body of evidence that suggests long-term cognitive issues with pediatric use of cannabinoids. Geriatric patients may be more sensitive to the sympathomimetic and psychoactive effects of Marinol. In addition, increased somnolence and dizziness may increase risk of falls. It is prudent to start at the lowest starting doses and titrate up very slowly.

Pregnant Women

Marinol has not been well studied in pregnant women. It is known that cannabinoids pass from the mother to the developing fetus. There is some low-quality scientific evidence that using cannabis during pregnancy may result in lower birth weight and neurologic deficits early on, and also later in childhood. Other studies suggest that babies exposed to cannabinoids *in utero* are at increased risk for asthma and other breathing issues. Marinol is placed in Category C for pregnancy risks. Based on studies in rodents, it should be used only if the potential benefits justify the potential risks.

Nursing Mothers

Marinol has not been studied in nursing mothers. A small study reported in 1990 suggested that cannabis exposure from breastfeeding in the first month of life could be associated with diminished motor development. Cannabinoids are fat soluble, so a very small percentage of the cannabinoids are passed to infants through to breast milk. However, the more a mother smokes, the higher the quantity of the cannabinoids in the breast milk. The American Academy of Pediatrics advises nursing mothers to abstain from using cannabis while breastfeeding.

PRECAUTIONS

Marinol may lower the seizure threshold. Seizure and seizure-like activity have been reported in patients taking Marinol. Marinol should be used with caution and close supervision in patients with a history of seizure disorder. Marinol should be discontinued if the patient develops seizures.

Because of the possibility of tachycardia, hypotension, hypertension, or syncope, Marinol should be used with caution in patients with cardiac disorders.

Psychiatric monitoring of patients on Marinol is recommended because of the possibility of the development of psychological and/or physiologic dependence. However, true addiction is uncommon. Marinol may aggravate pre-existing anxiety, depression, mania, or schizophrenia.

Patients concomitantly using CNS-depressant medications or alcohol may have additive or synergistic effects. These patients should be counseled about concomitant use of these.

Marinol may interfere with other medications via metabolic and pharmacodynamic mechanisms. It is highly protein-bound and may displace other protein-bound drugs. The patient should be monitored for changes in dosage requirements in patients taking concomitant highly protein-bound medications.

Otherwise, when it comes to issues related to abstinence syndrome, long-term use, psychosocial sequelae, carcinogenesis, mutagenesis, impairment of fertility and overdose, Marinol is very much like THC, discussed in Chapter 14.

NEWER, SUPERIOR MEDICATIONS
Since the discovery of far superior 5-HT3 (Zofran) and NK-1 (EMFND) antagonist medications for chemo-induced nausea and vomiting (CINV), there is little use for Marinol for this condition. Likewise, Megestrol has been shown to be superior to THC for weight gain in patients with cancer- and HIV-associated weight loss.

Cesamet
(www.webmd.com/drugs/2/drug-144710/cesamet-oral/details)
Cesamet (generic name: nabilone) is manufactured by Valeant Pharmaceuticals. It became available in 1985. It is FDA approved to treat chemotherapy-related nausea and vomiting (CINV) only in patients who have failed to respond adequately to conventional antiemetic treatments, due to its high rate of adverse side-effects. It is a synthetically manufactured cannabinoid, similar to THC, that comes in 1-mg capsules. It is FDA approved on Schedule II. It is believed to have a higher potential for abuse

than Marinol and has higher levels of psychoactive side-effects, requiring closer physician supervision.

INDICATIONS
Cesamet is used only to treat nausea and vomiting as chemotherapy-related side-effects if other antiemetic drugs have been ineffective.

DOSING
For chemotherapy-induced nausea and vomiting (CINV), the usual starting dose is 1 mg. The initial pre-chemotherapy dose should be given 1–3 hours before chemotherapy is administered. Then it should be taken three times a day during the entire course of chemotherapy. If the 1 mg dose is not effective, it can be gradually increased up to 2 mg three times a day.

Cesamet can be combined with other antiemetic medications, such as prochlorperazine, for additive effects and to decrease side-effects from higher doses of these medications if used alone.

In addition, because of a higher risk for psychological dependence, prescriptions for Cesamet should be limited to the number of doses necessary for a single cycle of chemotherapy.

SIDE-EFFECTS
Because it is essentially pure THC analogue, Cesamet can cause sympathomimetic side-effects such as tachycardia and conjunctival injection. Orthostatic hypotension has also been reported.

In addition, some patients report a dose-related "high" marked by outbursts of laughter, elation, and heightened awareness.

EFFICACY
Cesamet has dose-related effects on appetite, antiemetic effects, and psychoactive effects on cognition, memory, and perception. There is great patient-to-patient variation in response to the medication. Patients usually develop tolerance to the unpleasant side-effects of Cesamet within two weeks.

Cesamet is orally administered. It has an onset of action after 30–60 minutes and peak effect at 2–4 hours. There is a sizeable first-pass hepatic effect, and only 10–20 percent of the dose reaches the circulation. The psychoactive effects tend to last 4–6 hours, while the appetite-stimulation effect can last 24 hours or longer.

SPECIAL POPULATIONS

Pediatric and Geriatric Patients

Cesamet has not been studied in pediatric populations. Caution should be observed when using Cesamet in pediatric populations because of issues with its psychoactive effects. There is an increasing body of evidence that suggests long-term cognitive problems with pediatric use of cannabinoids. Geriatric patients may be more sensitive to the sympathomimetic and psychoactive effects of Cesamet. In addition, increased somnolence and dizziness may increase risk of falls. It is prudent to start at the lowest starting doses and titrate up very slowly.

Pregnant Women

Cesamet has not been well studied in pregnant women. It is Category C for pregnancy risks, based on studies in rodents. It should be used only if the potential benefits justify the potential risks. *See* the section on pregnant women in the previous discussion on Marinol in this chapter.

Nursing Mothers

Cesamet has not been studied in nursing mothers. *See* the section on nursing mothers in the previous discussion of Marinol above.

PRECAUTIONS

Cesamet may lower the seizure threshold. Seizure and seizure-like activity have been reported in patients taking Cesamet. Cesamet should be used with caution and close supervision in patients with a history of seizure disorder. Discontinue Cesamet if the patient develops seizures.

Because of the possibility of tachycardia, hypotension, hypertension, and syncope, the medication should be used with caution in patients with cardiac disorders.

Psychiatric monitoring of patients on Cesamet is recommended because of the possibility of the development of psychological and physiologic dependence. However, true addiction is uncommon. Cesamet may aggravate pre-existing anxiety, depression, mania, or schizophrenia.

Patients concomitantly using CNS-depressant medications or alcohol may have additive or synergistic effects. These patients should be counseled about concomitant use of these.

Cesamet may interfere with other medications via metabolic and pharmacodynamic mechanisms. It is highly protein-bound and may displace other protein-bound drugs. The patient should be monitored for changes in dosage requirements in patients taking concomitant highly protein-bound medications.

Otherwise, when it comes to issues related to abstinence syndrome, long-term use, psychosocial sequelae, carcinogenesis, mutagenesis, impairment of fertility and overdose, Cesamet is very much like THC, discussed in detail in Chapter 14.

NEWER, SUPERIOR MEDICATIONS

Since the discovery of far superior 5-HT3 (Zofran) and NK-1 (EMFND) antagonist medications for CINV, there is little use for Cesamet for this condition. Likewise, Megestrol has been shown to be superior to THC for weight gain in patients with cancer- and HIV-associated weight loss.

There are two new and promising plant-based cannabis medications, Sativex and Epidiolex, which are both made from extracts of plant material. As such, like the cannabis plant, they have combinations of THC, CBD, and terpenes. The results have been promising.

Sativex

(www.gwpharm.com/prescriberinformation.aspx)

Sativex (generic name: nabiximol) is manufactured by GW Pharmaceuticals. It is approved widely in Europe; it is also approved in Canada and other countries. Sativex has been used since 2010 making it the first plant-based prescription cannabis medication. Sativex is in Stage III trials to study its efficacy in treating cancer-related pain and MS-related spasticity.

It comes as a mouth spray made from naturally-occurring extracted oils from patented cannabis plants. It has a THC:CBD ratio of 1:1 and includes naturally occurring terpenes. Each spray delivers a fixed dose of 2.7 mg of THC and 2.5 mg of CBD. It is not yet FDA approved; however, it is currently being fast-tracked for treatment of patients with advanced cancer-related pain and treatment of MS spasticity. It is recommended for spasticity and neuropathic pain in MS patients. It has also shown promise for moderate to severe pain in cancer patients who are on the highest possible dose of opioids.

Sativex is well tolerated, due to the modifying effects of the CBD on the psychoactive effects of the THC. Possible side-effects included dizziness, disorientation, and drowsiness. About 12 percent of the patients in Phase III trials have stopped taking the medication due to side effects.

As with all preparations of cannabis medication, the proper dosing schedule has not been well defined.

Once Sativex becomes FDA approved, clinicians will be able to prescribe it, not just recommend it. In addition, the patient will be able to get this medication at community pharmacies and will not have to visit a medical dispensary. It should also be the first plant-based, natural cannabis medicine covered by health insurance for specific conditions.

Epidiolex
(www.gwpharm.com/prescriberinformation.aspx)
Epidiolex is manufactured by GW Pharmaceuticals. It is highly purified CBD from plant material. It is based on available limited studies, which have shown significant improvement in pediatric patients with intractable seizures when used as an oil or tincture. Epidiolex has been given orphan-drug designation for investigational new drug trials (IND) for Dravet and Lennox-Gastaut syndromes. It is also on the FDA's fast track for Dravet syndrome.

There are several other pharmaceuticals that are in various stages of clinical trials in the United States and Europe.

Caveat
The prescribing information in this chapter is current as of the date of publication of this book. The clinician is advised to read the current prescribing information provided by the manufacturer and Physician's Desk Reference (PDR).

HIV-related Wasting Syndrome

A patient has HIV-related wasting syndrome. He is extremely cachetic, and his specialist has been using Marinol for its appetite-stimulating effects. He has heard that plant-based cannabis is far superior to the pharmaceutical form of THC and wants to know what you think about Marinol versus plant-based cannabis.

Discussion: Marinol is a synthetically manufactured form of THC. As such, it does not contain any other cannabinoids such as CBD or terpenes. It has been used effectively to stimulate appetite and weight-gain for over two decades. It is available as oral capsules in a variety of doses. Because Marinol is pure THC without the balancing effects of CBD found in plant-based cannabis, it more commonly increases sympathomimetic effects, feelings of anxiety, and psychoactive effects than natural cannabis does. It can be much more costly than using plant-based medication, unless the cost of the Marinol is covered by health insurance.

Suggest to the patient that he talk with his specialist about the use of Marinol versus plant-based cannabis, which is often easier to titrate, and with fewer side-effects, than Marinol.

CHAPTER 6

Vehicles for Delivery and Routes of Administration

There is a variety of routes by which medical cannabis can be delivered; it can be inhaled by smoking or vaporizing it, ingested, or applied to the skin using dermal patches or creams. In addition, there is a wide variety of paraphernalia that has been designed over the years to deliver doses of the cannabinoids and assist with appropriate titration of the medicine. Cannabis-based medications are fat soluble so are usually inhaled or ingested. There is increasing research into means to more consistently administer the medicine transdermally.

The means by which cannabis is administered dramatically affects the onset of action, duration of action, clinical effects, and adverse effects.

Chapter 16 discusses how the clinician, caregiver, patient, and dispensary staff work together in selecting specific cultivars of cannabis, dosing, titrating, and choosing the best delivery vehicle for the patient's social and lifestyle needs.

The following text in this chapter summarizes what the clinician needs to know about current vehicles for delivery and means of administering medical cannabis.

Home-grown Cannabis Plants

It is important to have a working knowledge of how the drug can be purchased for use. Of course, the state laws allow for growing one's own cannabis plants. Seeds, growing materials, and training in cultivating one's own cannabis are usually easily available at dispensaries in states where medical cannabis is legal. The patient's caregiver can be assigned to cultivating cannabis plants for the patient's use. Home-grown plants can be used as dried buds, or the oils can be extracted in the kitchen to make cannabis butter for use in edibles.

Flowering Bud

Even with the many other means of administering cannabis, smoking is still by far the most common, even for medical use. Clinicians should be familiar with the fat, green, pungent cannabis bud which is the dried flower of the female cannabis plant. Over the past few decades, breeding of different cultivars of cannabis has focused on maximizing the percentage of THC and/or CBD in the bud.

There are literally hundreds of different cultivars of cannabis, with new ones being produced regularly. Some examples include BC Bud, Maui Wowie, Charlotte's Web, and White Widow. The cultivars are often named after the aromas given off by the terpenes in the bud or after the color of the cannabis resin glands, called *trichomes*. The smell and color of the hairs on the bud are not related to the potency of THC or CBD in the bud.

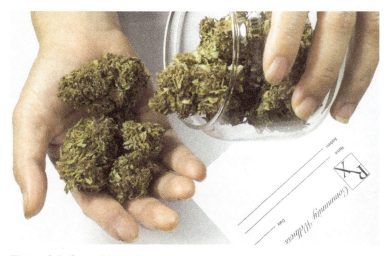

Figure 6-1 Cannabis bud

The different cultivars of cannabis displayed in dispensaries often have a label stating the percentages of THC and CBD. In general, there are three broad categories of bud. There are those with high-potency THC and low-potency CBD, those with approximately equal potency of THC and CBD, and those with high-potency CBD and very low-potency THC. The clinician and patient should be aware that the labels in the dispensaries stating the percentage of THC and CBD are notoriously inaccurate. Each new batch of bud may have markedly different potency, even if it came from the same dispensary and has the same cultivar. Because of this, the patient needs to evaluate each new batch of cannabis. As always, the therapeutic goal requires starting out with a low dose and titrating slowly up to reach the optimal clinical effect. The bud sold in recreational dispensaries, or for recreational purposes, tends to be very high in THC and low in CBD, which renders it of limited value for medical purposes.

Inhalation by Smoking or Vaporization

The bud can be smoked in rolling paper or in one of myriad glass, metal, wood, and water pipes, or it can be vaporized and inhaled using a large hand-held vaporizer. One inhalation of smoked or vaporized bud is referred to as a *hit* and provides approximately 50 milligrams of cannabinoid. The potency of the medical cannabis varies significantly: Lower potency medical cannabis usually requires three to five hits over 45 minutes to get the clinical effect, and more potent cultivars require one to two hits over 30 minutes. The effect usually lasts 1–2 hours.

The bud contains millions of tiny colored crystals. When the bud is heated up by a vaporizer or is burned, the crystals release a fume of medication that is inhaled. The THC and CBD are within the fume along with the vaporized terpenes. With smoked bud, the temperature gets much hotter than vaporized bud, and therefore hundreds of by-products of the burnt plant material are inhaled with the cannabinoids. Only about 12 percent of the gas content of the smoke is cannabinoids; the remainder is combusted by-products. These by-products can cause a temporary dry cough with inhalation. Long-term regular use of smoked cannabis can cause large-airway inflammation and chronic bronchitis symptoms. Some of the by-products in cannabis smoke are the same carcinogens found in tobacco

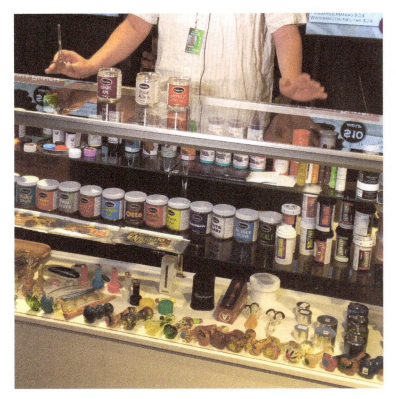

Figure 6-2 Various pipes available

smoke, including polycyclic aromatic hydrocarbons. However, the few available epidemiologic and clinical studies do not show an increased risk of airway cancer. It is postulated that the anti-cancer effects of the cannabinoids may be protective and mitigate against the risk of cancer. However, more high-quality studies need to be conducted on this subject before the cancer risk associated with smoking cannabis can be determined.

Larger, table-top vaporizers emit a stream of heated air to vaporize the cannabis plant material (leaf, wax, or oil). The smaller, hand-held devices that look like e-cigarettes have an atomizer that heats up the material. The vaporizers operate between 60 and 300 degrees Celsius. The temperature varies with the voltage, resistance, wetness of the material, and the contents of the liquid base that the material is in.

When using a vaporizer, about 95 percent of the vapor is cannabinoids, terpenes, and traces of carcinogenic polycyclic aromatic hydrocarbons (PAH). Also, there may be small amounts of organic pesticides or herbicides in the plant material.

Most of the larger, table-top vaporizers have the ability to control the temperature. The optimal setting is between 180–210 degrees Celsius (356–410 Fahrenheit). These temperatures produce maximum vaporization of the medically-important cannabinoids and terpenes with a minimum of other chemicals. Unfortunately, the hand-held vaporizers cannot control the temperature.

With vaporization there is no combustion, and therefore no by-products of combustion, as there are with smoked cannabis. The lack of combustion by-products make vaporization the preferable means of administering medical cannabis for patients with respiratory issues or for patients who have concerns about exposure to potential carcinogens.

The clinical effects of the medication are directly related to the amount of fume that the patient inhales. To maximize absorption of the medication from the fume in the alveolar gasses, the patient holds the inhaled fume in the lungs for several moments. About 95 percent of the cannabis in the fume is absorbed in the first few seconds. The patient is usually advised to start with one small, deep inhalation of the fume. The initial effects of the medication are usually any psychoactive effects; these can start in 5–15 minutes after the initial dose. The peak concentration of cannabinoids occurs in 2–10 minutes, declining rapidly over a period of 30 minutes, with only minimal generation of the other psychoactive metabolite, 11-OH-THC.

Depending on how the medication is working, the patient can continue to take small inhalations every 15–45 minutes to titrate up to the dose for the necessary clinical effect. Because the medication is inhaled and bypasses the liver, the first-pass effect that occurs with ingestion of cannabis is absent, and the onset of the clinical effect occurs much more quickly but also has a much shorter duration of action, 1–2 hours.

Smoking or vaporizing cannabis is most useful for a patient's episodic need for the medication for pain, spasms, seizures, decreased appetite, anxiety, or nausea and/or vomiting. Because inhaled cannabis medication has a rapid onset of action, a smoked or vaporized dose half an hour before bedtime is also superior for insomnia than a cannabis edible.

Smoking bud for medical purposes has several pitfalls. The first is the often-intense lingering aroma of the exhaled smoke. Since cannabis is still illegal in most states when used for non-medical purposes, this can lead to legal and social issues. Generally, the vaporized cannabis does not have nearly as much aroma as does smoked cannabis.

The second pitfall of smoking cannabis is that the smoke is made up of hundreds of by-products, some of which are known respiratory tract irritants. Clinicians wouldn't want to recommend use of smoked bud for patients with certain respiratory tract conditions or for use in and around children or other people with respiratory tract conditions.

Hashish

Hashish is made from the compressed colorful resin glands of the cannabis bud. It contains all of the same active ingredients as the bud, but it is more concentrated. Hashish is produced by extracting the cannabinoids with a solvent. The texture of hashish varies significantly, depending on how it is prepared. It can be hard and waxy, soft and pasty, or oily. The color ranges from earthy browns to tan and yellowish red. It has been around almost as long as humans have been smoking cannabis and has a long history of medical use.

Like the cannabis bud, hashish can be smoked or vaporized. It is titrated at the same intervals as smoked bud. However, it has a much higher concentration of cannabinoids and terpenes than cannabis bud, so the dose needs to be adjusted so as not to get too much medication with each inhalation. In general, hashish hits are about three times more potent than hits of cannabis bud, about 150 milligrams. Because hashish is mostly cannabinoid material, it has far fewer by-products of combustion, resulting in less respiratory tract irritation.

Cannabis bud and hashish are traditionally smoked or vaporized. There is very little available scientific evidence on the effects of second-hand smoke from cannabis preparations. However, there is anecdotal evidence to suggest that when there is very concentrated second-hand cannabis smoke or vapor in a closed environment, exposed non-smokers may experience psychoactive or physiologic effects from the medication. Of course, in this situation the exposed non-smoker would have a positive urine drug test for cannabinoids.[39]

Cannabis Oil

Cannabis oil is a highly concentrated form of cannabinoids in an oil base, made by solvent extraction. It is commonly known as *shatter* or *wax*. It can be green or greenish brown and has the consistency of soft wax. It usually comes in a potency of 60–85 percent cannabinoids, but it has been reported to contain as high as 99 percent cannabinoids. The oil can be consumed as an edible, but traditionally it is vaporized in a specially designed device for vaporization of the extract for inhalation. Cannabis oil is a formulation of THC most often used for recreational purposes. Most oils are produced locally and do not meet the high level of consistency and quality control that come with large-scale manufacturing. Cannabis oil formulations are very potent and are complex to administer, with a huge potential for causing extreme psychoactive effects. Therefore, it is not recommended for medical use.

Cannabis Tincture

Cannabis tinctures are alcohol extractions of all the active compounds in the cannabis plant. They contain very concentrated THC and CBD, but also all of the other organic chemicals in the plant. They may have an unpleasant taste and smell. Some extraction techniques minimize the amounts of terpenes and chlorophylls in the tincture. Most tinctures are produced locally and do not meet the high level of consistency and quality control that come with large-scale manufacturing.

Until cannabis was banned in 1937, pharmaceutical tinctures were the most commonly available cannabis medications. It is interesting to note in states where medical cannabis has been legal the longest, the trend has been away from smoked or vaporized cannabis and toward an increasing use of cannabis sold as a tincture or edible. This is because of the perceived negative effects of inhalation of cannabis, especially from smoking it, and associated social issues related to the aroma of the smoked or vaporized medicine.

Tinctures do not work as quickly as smoked or vaporized medicine, but they have a more rapid onset of action than other non-inhaled forms of the medicine. The tincture is a vehicle of approximately 75 percent alcohol delivered via a dropper under the tongue, where more rapid absorption occurs via sublingual arteries. The drug bypasses much of the liver's first-pass effect. Like the smoked or vaporized medicine, the tincture's onset of effects is quick and dissipates rapidly, in 1–2 hours.

In addition, the precise measurements afforded by a dropper and the precise concentrations of the tincture lead to consistent dosing for the patient. It is important to advise the patient not to swallow the preparation, as this will cause it to pass through the gastrointestinal tract and be subject to the liver's first-pass effect. If the tincture is added to a tea or liquid, then it is absorbed as an edible form of the medication, with the slow and gradual onset of effect associated with all cannabinoids that go through the gastrointestinal system.

The type of cannabinoids present (THC and/or CBD) and their concentrations will be documented on the tincture packaging. Like strains of cannabis, these concentrations are often incorrect if the product does not have high standards of preparation and quality control.

Cannabis Butter and Other Edibles

Cannabis butter is a soft, light green substance with a buttery texture. It is made by cooking cannabis bud in butter to extract the cannabinoids into the butter. It is seldom eaten by itself but is used to cook and bake a wide variety of cannabis edibles.

In addition to baked goods such as brownies, cookies, and cupcakes, there is an increasing variety of candies, chocolates, and flavored drinks that contain extracted cannabinoids. The dose of THC, and sometimes CBD, is documented on the label in milligrams, but again, the amounts given on the labels are notoriously inaccurate. Fortunately, the inaccuracy is usually in *overestimating* the amount of cannabinoids, but not always.

The cannabinoids in edibles are digested in the gastrointestinal tract and are thus subject to the liver's first-pass effect. This causes the onset of action to be much longer, about 1–2 hours, and the effects to last much longer, 5–6 hours. In addition, when THC is ingested and metabolized by the liver, it is actually converted to a different substance called *11-OH-THC*. This has a very strong affinity for CB1 receptors and it is 10 times more psychoactive than delta-9-THC or delta-8-THC, which are in inhaled cannabis.

Use of cannabis butter and other cannabis edibles has several benefits. They have a slow onset of action, and prolonged duration of effect, making them good for chronic pain control and night-time dosing.

Edibles are hard to dose because of the large variation in the batches produced in small manufacturing operations. Also, the amount of active ingredients in edibles decreases with longer duration of exposure to stomach acids. The presence or absence of food in the stomach can likewise affect absorption and clinical effects.

Like all products available in cannabis dispensaries, the amount of THC and CBD documented on the labels of edible products may be incorrect due to problems with quality control and their manufacturing in small start-up companies that make them. Once again, when dosing and titrating, the patient should start with a low dose—a small piece of the edible—and increase the amount slowly until he or she feels comfortable that the correct dose for the condition has been achieved.

Edibles can be hard to titrate because of the slow onset of action and long duration of effect, and as previously stated, there is often markedly less cannabinoid in the product than the label says. There are few standards for labeling and packaging of these products. A recent informal analysis of several popular brands of edibles in Colorado found that for almost all of the products sold by several manufacturers, only a minute fraction of the cannabinoid content stated on the label was actually present.

In time, new regulations and enforcement will result in higher quality and standards for edibles. However, for the present time, the patient will have to become familiar with how to dose different brands of edibles.

A safety issue related to cannabis edibles has been recognized. The products usually come in attractive packaging and are usually tasty treats such as baked goods, candies, or soft drinks. This has resulted in a spike in the number of children mistakenly ingesting these edibles and ending up in the emergency room. There are no reported deaths, but serious side-effects from the psychoactive effects have been reported. New laws are being enacted to mandate packaging standards and require single-wrap servings to prevent accidental excessive dosing.

Cannabis edibles are popular with patients because, like tinctures, they do not involve smoke or vapor, so there is no tell-tale smell or respiratory tract irritation. In addition, they can be ingested anywhere and are reasonably priced, compared to cannabis bud or hashish.

Cannabis Creams or Lotions

Creams, ointments, and lotions are probably the oldest vehicles for delivering cannabis, going back thousands of years. These have cannabis oil in them. Unlike the dermal patches, described below, these products are absorbed only superficially into the local area. They are used for localized arthritis, dermatitis, psoriasis, or severely dry skin. There is little research supporting these uses, so it is not clear how much of the cannabinoids are actually absorbed into the skin. However, thousands of years of anecdotal observation, and the fact that THC and CBD have anti-inflammatory effects at a cellular level and capsaicin-like effects on the TRPV-1 receptors, suggest that transdermal delivery may be a reasonable treatment option. With this route of administration, there is minimal absorption into the bloodstream, and therefore no, or minimal, psychoactive effects. In addition, these topical formulations can be combined with topical anti-fungals or antibiotics to also treat fungal or bacterial skin infections.

Dermal Patches

Dermal patches are the newest vehicles for delivery of medical cannabis. Much like nicotine patches, they are formulated so that they can be worn on the skin to gradually release a dose into the body, usually 10 mg or 20 mg of cannabinoids, through dermal absorption over several hours. Usually they can be applied to any area of the body with good circulation. The skin is prepped with an isopropyl alcohol swab to disinfect and facilitate the transfer of the medicine. The cannabinoids go directly into the blood stream, like smoked or vaporized cannabis. The dermal patches release the cannabinoids gradually, creating a sustained effect for 8–12 hours. The effects start within 15–30 minutes. The patches can be cut smaller to adjust the dose. Skin irritation can occur with repeated use, so the patch application site should be varied to prevent this adverse effect.

Only a few medical patches are currently available. They come in a variety of formulations, with various CBD to THC ratios. There are also patches with isolated CBD or CBN.

Over-the-Counter CBD Oil

CBD oil that was obtained from hemp plants is legal and available over-the-counter in many states. The patient can buy the CBD oil for a vaporizer at many e-cigarette stores. This oil is produced using the legal industrial hemp seeds and stems. This is based on a federal court case that stated the DEA "cannot regulate naturally-occurring CBD not contained within or derived from" non-psychoactive hemp not included in Schedule I".[4]

CBD oil usually comes in 1.3 mg to 3.0 mg per milliliter concentrations in 10–20 ml vials. Hemp is extremely low in CBD, about 25 parts per million, but large scale manufacturers in Europe are able extract the CBD for this use. Because illegal strains of cannabis were not used to obtain the oil, it is legal in many states and sold as a food additive. This oil is generally used in a vaporizer, but it could be ingested in an edible as well.

Calculating the Dose of Inhaled Cannabis

There is slightly less than 500 milligrams of cannabis in an average size joint. One ounce is 28 grams, so there are approximately 60 joints in 1 ounce of cannabis. A typical dose is 3 to 5 hits, or 100–200 milligrams of cannabis material, about one-third to one-half of a joint. Experimenting with low doses and slow titration of smoked or vaporized cannabis is always recommended. The common mistake is for the patient to not feel enough of an effect after only a few minutes and then take another hit of the medicine. This can lead to excessive psychoactive effects and to anxiety and nausea.

If the clinician wants to be specific with the number of milligrams of medication that the patient will be receiving, he or she will need to know the potency of the plant material.

If it takes half of a joint for the patient to get the desired effects, based on the averages, we can estimate how many

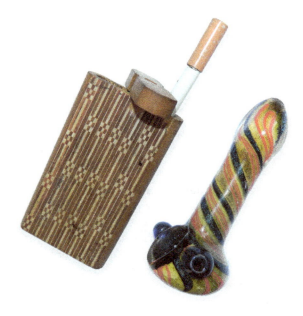

Figure 6-3 Examples of a pipe, at left; glass bowl, at right

milligrams of THC that would be. One half of a joint would be about 200 mg of dried cannabis plant material. So 200 mg of dry herb x 15% THC potency = 30 mg total THC. Because of the nature of smoking, about 25 percent of that is actually absorbed into the blood stream. So, in this scenario 30 mg x 25% = avg. 7.5 mg of THC is inhaled. Ingested cannabis affects the body differently than smoked cannabis so the patient shouldn't expect an identical effect as that from smoking cannabis if he or she ingests an identical amount of oral medicine, but it's a safe reference point to get started.

The plant material can be rolled in a cigar wrapper called a *blunt*. However, usually, this requires a considerable amount of the material, 500–1000 mg, and much more than one patient would require for a dose. It is not recommended for medical use.

The plant material can also be smoked in a pipe or glass bowl. As long as a small size pipe or bowl is used, the amount of plant material and dosing can be easily regulated by the patient. Large and very large pipes and bowls are available, for use by groups of people recreationally, but these are not recommended for medical use.

The plant materials, bud or hashish, as well as the oil and tinctures, can all be vaporized by large-table top devices and the newer handheld vaporizers, as previously discussed. The dose of cannabinoids from a vaporizer is the same as for smoked dried-cannabis plant material.

CLINICAL SCENARIO

Debilitating Back Pain and Best Route of Administration

The symptoms of a patient with intermittent episodes of debilitating back pain have been well controlled for over a year. He uses medical cannabis a few times a month for flare-ups of pain and spasm. He wants to know which is the best route of administration for this condition. What do you tell him?

Discussion: In this scenario the patient needs to use the medicine only a few times a month. The episodes are painful and debilitating and the patient would like immediate relief. Ask if the patient will be able to rest and abstain from driving or activities that would be dangerous if he has significant psychoactive side-effects from the batch of cannabis that he uses. He will need to titrate the medication over 30–45 minutes to get relief. Vaporized or smoked cannabis would provide rapid onset of relief in a few minutes of the initial dose. The amount and frequency of doses can be modified to control the pain and spasm, while minimizing the psychoactive effects. The effects of the smoked or vaporized cannabis will wear off in 1–2 hours, allowing for quick return to normal function as the flare-up eases off. The cannabis can be stored long term, for easy use, when necessary.

PART II

Conditions and Symptoms

CHAPTER 7

Qualifying Conditions Under Current Laws

Federal Law

As of the date of this book's publication, no cannabis plants are legal under Federal law.

However, the Compassionate Access, Research Expansion, and Respect States Act of 2015 (CARERS) was introduced in the U.S. Senate in March of 2015. It has yet to be voted on. This bill amends the Controlled Substances Act (CSA) to move cannabis from Schedule I to Schedule II.

Other provisions of the Act are:
- It excludes CBD, when used alone, from the definition of cannabis.
- It attempts to fix the problem with federal banking laws that have restrictions related to cannabis-related monies. Currently all dispensaries are on a "cash only" basis, due to banking laws and federally illegal drugs.
- It terminates the very restrictive federal "Guidance on Procedures for the Provision of Marijuana for Medical Research" (issued on May 21, 1999), which has severely limited clinical research on the medical effects of cannabis.
- It rescinds the University of Mississippi's monopoly for the growing and manufacturing of cannabis and cannabis derivatives for research purposes.
- It allows Veterans Administration health care providers to write recommendations for cannabis in states with medical cannabis laws.

This bill has bipartisan support and has progressed well since its legislative introduction, but it has not yet been enacted as law. If CARERS is enacted as law, medical cannabis will immediately become legal throughout the United States and the U.S. Territories.

State and Jurisdictional Laws

As of October 2015, 23 states and the District of Columbia (DC) have some sort of legalized medical and/or recreational cannabis laws. Some states have limited CBD-only laws. Eleven (11) other states are in the process of enacting, or are likely to enact, medical and/or recreational cannabis laws by the November 2016 election.

From the original medical cannabis initiative, California's Proposition 215 enacted as law in 1996, until Florida's recent attempt to pass in 2014, the original concept behind state legislation to legalize medical cannabis was that it would be used only for patients with severe, chronic, and debilitating diseases or conditions who had already had maximum therapy with generally accepted medications yet were still quite symptomatic. It is not uncommon, however, for state legislation to have additional text similar to California's: "or any other illness for which marijuana provides relief," again if the patient is severely debilitated.

The founding idea behind each state law is that medical cannabis would be used as an adjunct to other standard treatments for the specific qualifying conditions. In addition, when these laws were drafted, it was expected that because of the severity of the debilitating conditions of patients who qualified for medical cannabis, many of them would require a medical caregiver to help them grow or obtain cannabis plant material.

As is typical of medical practice dictated by political agenda rather than research, there is very little high-quality evidence to support any of the qualifying conditions in the various states' legislation. It is not that medical cannabis isn't helpful or palliative for these and other conditions, but more the lack of quality research on the subject.

The qualifying conditions vary significantly from state to state, often based on anecdotal experience or emotional outcries from a vociferous few, owing to the lack of solid scientific research. In time, the state-specific qualifying conditions will, no doubt, be amended and expanded. Because of the distinct possibility that medical cannabis will be moved from Schedule I to Schedule II in the near future, the states' lists of qualifying conditions will probably become irrelevant in clinical practice.

State-specific qualifying conditions, as of the publication of this book, are:

- Anorexia/cachexia
- Arthritis
- Cancer
- Chronic pain
- Crohn's disease
- Glaucoma
- HIV/AIDS
- Migraines
- Multiple sclerosis (MS)
- Parkinson's disease
- Post-traumatic stress disorder (PTSD)
- Seizures
- Spasticity/muscle spasms

The website www.MedicalMarijuana.procon.org provides up-to-date details on the status of each state that has legalized medical cannabis. The website also maintains a current state-by-state list of "approved" or "qualifying" medical conditions and information about patient registration requirements and fees. Additionally, each state medical board maintains this information. Each state's list of qualifying medical conditions is constantly subject to change for these states. In general, the medical board for each state or jurisdiction where medical cannabis is legal has a policy statement outlining standards of good practice.

In addition, each state law provides for protection of clinicians from criminal or civil liability for recommending or approving the medicinal use of cannabis by a patient if there is a bona fide physician-patient relationship. Clinicians are allowed to openly discuss the medical use of cannabis with a patient. Clinicians who provide cannabis to patients or direct patients where to procure cannabis are not protected. Only Montana and Oregon allow out-of-state patients to obtain medical cannabis. In all states, only the physician can "authorize" the recommendation letter. However, in general, mid-level providers can do the evaluation of the patient prior to the physician's consideration of authorization.

STATES AND DISTRICT OF COLUMBIA

Restrictions
See Appendix A, which lists specific restrictions on the use of medical cannabis.

Training Requirements
Most states do not have a training or continuing medical education (CME) requirement prior to recommending medical cannabis.

- **Alaska:** No specific training or CME required.
- **Arizona:** No specific training or CME required. The Arizona Department of Health Services has collaborated with the University of Arizona's Mel and Enid Zuckerman College of Public Health to develop a free 5-hour online CME course on the physician's role and expectations under the Arizona Medical Marijuana Program. However, this is not a requirement.
- **California:** No specific training or CME required. The University of California at San Francisco has robust educational and CME offerings.
- **Colorado:** No specific training or CME required. The Colorado medical board is currently considering drafting a policy on the use of cannabis as a therapeutic option.
- **Connecticut:** No specific training or CME required. Yale University offers a 1-hour CME course entitled "Risk Management and Understanding the Prescribing Process of Medical Marijuana."
- **Delaware:** No specific training or CME required. However, the Delaware Marijuana Program specifically stipulates that CME resources should be developed to teach physicians about medical cannabis.
- **District of Columbia:** No specific training or CME required.

- **Florida:** Has recently passed a CBD law. This requires an 8-hour CME training course prior to recommending CBD. The Florida Medical Association and Florida Osteopathic Association sponsor the required CME. The state's qualifying medical conditions are very restrictive.
- **Georgia:** No specific training or CME required. The state has recently passed a CBD law. The medical board policy is still being drafted.
- **Hawaii:** No specific training or CME required.
- **Illinois:** No specific training or CME required.
- **Maine:** No specific training or CME required. The Maine Medical Association has a CME video to help physicians understand the state's medical cannabis law.
- **Maryland:** No specific training or CME required.
- **Massachusetts:** Physicians who certify patients for medical cannabis must first complete the Massachusetts Medical Society's 2-hour CME course on the clinical and legal aspects of the state's medical cannabis law.
- **Michigan:** No specific training or CME required.
- **Minnesota:** No specific training or CME required. The Minnesota Medical Association has developed a webinar for physician training on medical cannabis.
- **Montana:** No specific training or CME required.
- **Nevada:** No specific training or CME required.
- **New Hampshire:** No specific training or CME required.
- **New Jersey:** No specific training or CME required.
- **New Mexico:** No specific training or CME required.
- **New York:** 4.0 hour online CME course required by Medical Board.
- **Oregon:** No specific training or CME required.
- **Rhode Island:** No specific training or CME required.
- **Vermont:** No specific training or CME required.
- **Washington:** No specific training or CME required.

U.S. TERRITORIES
- **Guam:** In November 2014, the voters of Guam approved a ballot initiation legalizing medical cannabis for debilitating medical conditions.

- **Puerto Rico:** In May 2015, the Governor signed an executive order that legalized cannabis for medical purposes. Rules and regulations were expected by October 2015.

Canada

Unlike the United States, where there is a patchwork of laws from state to state, cannabis is federally regulated and uniform across Canada. In June 2015, the Supreme Court of Canada allowed the use of medical cannabis material beyond that of smokeable dried cannabis bud, i.e., edibles, concentrates, and topical lotions.

As in the United States, clinicians do not write a prescription for cannabis but instead produce a "medical document" recommending it. This document is then taken to the dispensary, where a lengthy verification process occurs between the dispensary and the recommending clinician. Because of Canada's insurance laws, clinicians cannot bill for patient evaluation and treatment with medical cannabis. It is estimated that there are currently only about 37,000 Canadians using this onerous system to get medical cannabis. However, laws enacted in spring 2015 are expected to dramatically increase the size of the medical cannabis market throughout Canada.

There has been strong federal opposition against the expansion of recreational or medical cannabis from the previous conservative Canadian government. It is expected that the new liberal government will likely legalize recreational cannabis.

The Canadian Medical Association has developed several online CME courses on medical cannabis practice and laws.

CHAPTER 8

Conditions and Symptoms Responsive to Medical Cannabis

Research and clinical studies and anecdotal reports that support the efficacy of medical cannabis for treating the qualifying conditions, as well as some other conditions and symptoms, are discussed in this chapter. It is important to juxtapose the qualifying conditions, as determined by state legislatures, with the actual research findings. There is an excellent review of the peer-reviewed literature for the period 1990–2014 from the organization ProCon.org (http://medicalmarijuana. procon.org/view.resource.php?resourceID=000884). This concise analysis looked at the 60 available peer-review studies on cannabis used for medical purposes to treat symptoms and medical conditions. It briefly summarizes whether the studies' findings support the efficacy of medical cannabis for each condition. There was a total of 15 conditions and symptoms for which sufficient studies were available. Although there were several good studies of CBD alone for treatment of epilepsy and seizures, dystonia, and spasm that were available during this time period, unfortunately they were not discussed.

Research findings on medical cannabis for glaucoma were not clearly pro or con, but there are already far superior pharmaceuticals for this condition.

Findings of 11 studies supported use of medical cannabis for multiple sclerosis (MS); however, those of four did not, and those of four others were inconclusive.

Of the total of 60 studies, findings of only one study (one of six studies of HIV) showed no medical benefit of cannabis. This single study showed that smoking cannabis contributed to pulmonary symptoms due to the irritants in the smoke and did not recommend its use in HIV patients. The other five studies of HIV showed that cannabis was beneficial for pain relief and stimulation of appetite.

The other studies were all supportive of medical benefits for cannabis in amyotrophic lateral sclerosis (ALS), bipolar disorder, cancer, Huntington's disease, inflammatory bowel disease (IBD)/Crohn's, nausea, pain, Parkinson's disease, post-traumatic stress disorder (PTSD), psychosis/schizophrenia, rheumatoid arthritis, and Tourette syndrome.

In all of the studies, cannabis was an adjunct medication used for symptoms associated with the condition, such as anxiety, pain, inflammation, insomnia, poor appetite, and nausea and vomiting.

Much of the legislation that has been passed is highly biased and not scientifically based. It is the paucity of good scientific data due to cannabis's classification as a Schedule I substance for 40 years that has created this dearth of good scientific evidence. For example, New York State became the 23rd state to legalize medical cannabis in 2014; however, the law doesn't allow for smoked cannabis. If the research were going to support any form of cannabis, then smoked and vaporized plant material would have to be considered the most efficacious, except in patients with pulmonary conditions. Indeed, the two FDA-approved cannabinoid pharmaceuticals are the least effective and have the greatest side-effects. It is the entourage effect of THC, CBD, and probably the other cannabinoids and terpenes present in plant material that makes cannabis efficacious, with a low-side-effect profile.

Specifics on studies that have been conducted to determine the efficacy and side-effects of medical cannabis for specific symptoms and conditions are discussed below.

Chronic Pain

By far, pain is the most common symptom for which a patient seeks medical cannabis: up to 94 percent of patients in Colorado and about 85 percent of patients in Michigan.

In Montréal, Canada, where medical marijuana has been available for years, about 10–15 percent of patients attending chronic pain clinics use cannabis as part of their pain management.

There is a shortage of pain management specialists, and most chronic pain conditions will be managed, in the long term, by primary care clinicians. A recent study by the American Academy of Family Physicians found significant, widespread deficits among primary care physicians in the medical knowledge and skills necessary for providing optimal pain management, reducing medication risks, and evaluating addictive behaviors (http://www.aafp.org/patient-care/public-health/pain-opioids.html).

Over the past two decades, chronic pain has become an epidemic in the United States. The National Centers for Health Statistics estimates that as many as 80 million people suffer from chronic pain—more than the number of people with heart disease, diabetes and cancer, combined. The economic and social impact of disability from pain, and from the secondary effects of the medications used to treat pain, is enormous and growing.

As discussed in previous chapters, cannabis has been shown to be effective for a variety of pain conditions, including neuropathic, myopathic, and arthritic pain. In addition, it relieves muscle stiffness, spasm, and inflammation and alleviates anxiety and depressed mood, which often accompany chronic pain.[40,41]

A study of intractable neurogenic pain from a variety of causes, including multiple sclerosis, brachial plexus injury, limb amputation, and spinal cord injury, found that cannabidiol (CBD) resulted in superior pain relief, compared to placebo, without side-effects.[42] However, with cancer patients there was no significant pain reduction with CBD alone.[43]

As of May 2014, the Center for Medicinal Cannabis Research at University of California campuses had completed 13 approved studies. Of those, seven were published double-blind, placebo-controlled studies that evaluated pain relief, and each showed cannabis to be effective.

In general, as with all conditions for which medical cannabis is used, it is not the primary treatment for chronic pain conditions but is an adjuvant treatment to consider. As discussed at the end of this chapter, cannabis can be effectively used to decrease or discontinue opioid use in patients who wish or need to decrease addictive and dangerous oral opioids.[44]

HOW CANNABIS REDUCES PAIN

The available studies show that, much like opioid receptors, increased levels of CB1 receptors are found in regions of the brain that regulate nociceptive processing. In addition, cannabinoids may contribute to pain modulation through anti-inflammatory mechanisms. On mast cells, CB2 receptors attenuate the release of inflammatory agents such as histamine and serotonin. Studies show cannabinoids are synergistic with opioids in reducing the nociceptive response. One study reported that the efficacy of synthetic CB1- and CB2-receptor agonists were comparable with the efficacy of morphine in a murine model of tumor pain.[40,41]

In general, cannabis is much safer than either nonsteroidal anti-inflammatory drugs (NSAIDs) or opioid pain medications, and has fewer side-effects, a much lower risk for dependence than opioids, and a huge therapeutic window compared to opioids. This allows for the patient to gradually titrate to the right dose, with the right delivery vehicle to get modest to marked pain relief. In addition, about one-third of chronic pain patients develop anxiety secondary to the condition causing the pain. These patients are often on a benzodiazepine as well as an opioid. In carefully selected patients, cannabis has a separate and distinct effect in reducing anxiety. Medical cannabis patients who do develop dependence are much easier to manage than those with opioid or benzodiazepine dependence.

STARTING A PATIENT WITH PAIN ON MEDICAL CANNABIS

Starting a patient on medical cannabis for pain is fairly complicated, and a number of preferable alternatives are available for acute and subacute pain, so *it is recommended that cannabis be recommended only for use by patients with chronic pain conditions.*

Chronic pain is persistent and often worsens. By definition, its duration is 12 weeks or more, often lasting many months or years. It may initially start in response to an injury or surgery, but the pain continues long after the tissues have healed. This is in contrast to acute pain or sub-acute pain, which occurs suddenly in response to an injury, surgery, or flare-up of a condition but abates within weeks to several months. The goal of treatment for chronic pain is to reduce symptoms and improve function.

Cannabis can be used alone to obtain pain relief or in combination with generally-recognized opioid and NSAID analgesics.

In addition to its specific pain-relieving effects, cannabis often has a sedating effect and relieves anxiety, resulting in improved sleeping, and fewer sleep disturbances attributable to the pain.

CENTRAL PAIN

Centrally-mediated pain includes some forms of paresthesias, numbness, and burning sensations. The American Academy of Neurology reviewed the available literature, and based on the "highest quality evidence" considering "safety and effectiveness," determined that CBD can help lessen central pain (https://www.aan.com/Guidelines/home/GetGuidelineContent/650).

NEUROPATHIC PAIN

Chronic neuropathic pain accounts for 25–50 percent of all pain clinic visits. Diabetic peripheral neuropathy is the most common cause; this is related to the current diabetes epidemic in the United States. There are only a small number of FDA-approved medications specifically for neuropathic pain, and often opioids are also prescribed to help the patient tolerate uncontrolled pain.

Recently, several high-quality studies of chronic neuropathic pain have been done. These showed a moderate therapeutic effect from inhaled doses of cannabis. Two recent randomized, placebo-controlled clinical trials of neuropathic pain in HIV patients showed that inhaled cannabis reduced pain by 30 percent compared to placebo.[40] A 2013 study showed that low-dose vaporized cannabis (1.29 percent THC) resulted in 30 percent reduction of neuropathic pain in patients already being treated with conventional medications. The low-dose vaporized cannabis resulted in minimal psychoactive and cognitive deficits and was as effective as a high-dose (3.53 percent THC) of inhaled cannabis.[41] Other high-quality studies comparing high- to low-dose vaporized cannabis are currently being conducted to determine their efficacy in treating patients with chronic regional pain syndrome (CRPS,) post-herpetic neuralgia, spinal cord injury, or multiple sclerosis.

Other double-blind, randomized placebo-controlled studies have shown that cannabis significantly alleviated neuropathic pain by decreasing pain sensitivity and increasing pain tolerance.[46]

SYMPATHETIC PAIN

Chronic regional pain syndrome (CRPS) and the other sympathetically-mediated pain syndromes cause the most severe intractable pain. In addition to high doses of fast- and slow-release opioids, patients with CRPS often end up with surgically implanted spinal cord stimulators or opioid pumps. Currently, there are no studies to support recommending medical cannabis for these patients. However, empirical evidence and the inherent safety of well-managed use of cannabis suggest that oral formulations of high-CBD and low- or medium-potency THC medicine should have positive clinical effects for the neuropathic pain, spasticity, and sleep disturbance that accompany CRPS.

ARTHRITIS PAIN

Cannabis that contains both THC and CBD has several mechanisms of action for arthritis pain sufferers. In addition to the central-pain-relieving effects of THC, CBD has peripheral anti-inflammatory effects, and both cannabinoids help to improve sleep onset in pain sufferers. However, in general, the clinical benefits for patients with arthritis are felt to be modest, underscoring the use of medical cannabis as adjuvant therapy, in addition to traditional arthritis medications. However, two large-scale surveys in the United Kingdom and Australia indicated that about one-third of people using medical cannabis do so for arthritic pain, and most report considerable pain relief.[47]

In the last decade, a small well-designed study of rheumatoid arthritis patients showed that Sativex, the cannabis-based oromucosal spray, resulted in small but statistically significant improvements in pain on movement, pain at rest, and quality of sleep. There was no effect on morning stiffness. The side-effects were mild to moderate in nature. Additional studies were recommended.[48]

A study published in *Biological and Pharmaceutical Bulletin* showed that several different cannabinoids inhibit COX-2 enzyme activity.[49]

FIBROMYALGIA

A recent Canadian study of 457 patients with fibromyalgia showed that 13 percent used cannabis to manage their symptoms. The new *Canadian Fibromyalgia Treatment Guideline* states that cannabis should be considered for fibromyalgia patients with sleep disturbance.[50]

CHRONIC MYOFASCIAL PAIN

It is important to note that, in general, medical cannabis is indicated as adjuvant therapy for chronic pain conditions, although acute and subacute myofascial pain, associated with an injury or surgery, is better managed with short-term use of NSAIDs and/or opioids. Chronic myofascial pain that is not well managed with other medications, exercise, trigger point injections, and massage may respond to a trial of cannabis. Edible cannabis is usually preferred for its long half-life. However, if there are episodes of breakthrough pain, smoked or vaporized cannabis can be slowly titrated until a therapeutic effect is achieved.

MIGRAINE HEADACHES

Migraine headaches are commonly seen in primary practice. They usually present with unilateral or bilateral throbbing temporal pain, nausea, vomiting, and photosensitivity. They are vascular in nature.

Migraine headaches are considered a qualifying condition in some states, and anecdotal reports suggest cannabis may be beneficial for these types of headaches. Cannabis can have a positive therapeutic effect on the pain, and nausea and vomiting. However, because the underlying pain is due to vasodilation, and cannabis contributes to further cerebral vasodilation, it may not be a good treatment. It is not recommended at this time.

OPIOIDS AND CANNABIS

Patients using opioids for chronic pain often become tolerant of the opioid dose, resulting in a gradual escalation of the dose and the frequency of use. In addition, opioid overdose is an ever-increasing problem in our society. The death rate for opioid overdose quadrupled from 1999 to 2011, with 11,700 reported deaths due to semi-synthetic opioid-analgesic poisoning in 2011.[51] In one-third of the opioid deaths, there was concomitant use of a benzodiazepine, leading to a lethal drug-drug interaction. The recent changes in state and federal laws has slowed the mortality rate in recent years.

There is plenty of empirical evidence that for patients using opioids, the introduction of cannabis can lead to the gradual decrease or, in some cases, discontinuation of opioids for pain management. In addition, self-report surveys show that the common side-effects of opioid use, such as depression, constipation and nausea, were reduced with concomitant use of cannabis.[52] Unfortunately, high-quality studies of this have not yet been conducted.

However, a well-conducted epidemiologic study done during the period 1999–2010 showed a 25 percent lower rate of lethal opioid overdose in states with medical cannabis laws.

The rate decreased over time, after the enactment of state legalization as law. This would be the equivalent of 4,000 fewer deaths annually if this rate of decrease in opioid-related deaths had occurred in all 50 states.[53]

One recent small study showed that in patients using long-acting morphine or oxycodone, the addition of vaporized cannabis resulted in significant additional decreases in measured pain levels.[54] This finding suggests that cannabis may potentiate the pain-relieving effects of opioids, which could result in decreased use of opioid medication. The anti-anxiety effects of cannabis can also be used to reduce or discontinue the concomitant use of benzodiazepines. In addition, the anti-nausea effects of cannabis are often useful for patients taking opioids.

A recent study of CBD, in combination with morphine, showed a synergistic effect on nociceptive pain, suggesting that CBD may have promise as an opioid-sparing agent.[42]

If a patient is already taking opioids for chronic pain and does not have adequate control of the pain or wishes to taper off opioids, a trial of cannabis is appropriate. The most common adverse effects from inhaled or edible cannabis are the psychoactive effects, and the available studies suggest that the pain-relieving effects of cannabis occur at low doses. These low doses would be associated with little or no psychoactive effects.

A 2010 clinical study conducted at San Francisco General Hospital evaluated 24 patients using morphine or oxycodone for chronic pain.[55] The clinicians continued the opioids and added three daily doses of vaporized cannabis. This measurably improved pain control, and the "high" associated with the cannabis use gradually decreased to 1/10th of the original level within three to five days of use, but the pain-relieving effects continued. Pain levels were reduced an additional 33–44 percent with ongoing use of cannabis plus the opioid. Further study of higher doses or more frequent administration of vaporized or edible cannabis was recommended.

SAFETY ISSUES

As discussed in previous chapters, cannabis has very few long-term side-effects in adults; after they learn how to titrate medical cannabis, most of the psychoactive side-effects dissipate. Patients at risk for psychotic episodes can be screened out, and use of cannabis discontinued early if these episodes occur. There are few long-term side-effects other than the approximately 11 percent of patients who develop psychological and possibly physical dependence. These patients can also be identified early and managed appropriately.

It is probably impossible to overdose on cannabis. This is because there are no endocannabinoid receptors in the midbrain respiratory centers. Therefore, very high doses of THC or CBD do not cause fatal respiratory depression. According to a 2009 study published in *American Scientist*, a person would probably need 1,000 times the effective dose of cannabis for it to possibly be fatal. That being said, there have been numerous reports of the psychoactive effects of cannabis contributing to death by accidents.[45]

TREATMENT RECOMMENDATIONS

The empirical evidence suggests that long-acting oral preparations of cannabis are optimal for suppression of chronic pain. This is analogous to the use of slow-release opioids. Patients with continuous pain often prefer an edible form of cannabis because of its much longer half-life and the all-night duration of a bedtime dose. The active metabolite of edible THC is 11-OH-THC, which is 10 times more potent than inhaled THC.

It is recommended that inhaled cannabis be used initially as a trial form of the drug to determine efficacy, dose, and adverse effects. If there is a positive response to the use of inhaled cannabis, estimated equivalent doses of edible cannabis can be tried. Usually the pain can be controlled with slow-release oral preparations, and intermittent inhalations of vaporized or smoked cannabis can be used to control breakthrough or episodic flare-ups of pain.

For a patient seeking to use cannabis to control chronic pain, it is recommended that cannabis with approximately equal proportions of THC and CBD be used. The initial trial should use a vaporized or smoked dose. As always with cannabis medications, start low and titrate up slowly. Since the pain- and spasm-relieving effects of cannabis occur at low doses, the occurrence of psychoactive effects suggests that the patient has inhaled more medication than necessary. This is especially true after cannabis has been used for several days. The doses should initially be three times a day, and they should be slowly increased in frequency if necessary.

If the patient is using concomitant pain-relieving medications, efforts should be made to gradually decrease the dosing frequency of them with the use of adjuvant cannabis. At the follow-up visits, the clinician can review the pain diary and discuss the pain pattern and any changes in the use of other medications. Lowering the doses of the other medications can be considered after detailed consideration of the potential for, and possible consequences of, opioid withdrawal.

Cannabis can have a significant impact on pain-related anxiety, often reducing it, but increasing it in a small percentage of cannabis users. (*See* page 86 for a discussion of anxiety and cannabis use.) Because of the high proportion of chronic pain patients who also take benzodiazepines, the clinician should assess the impact of cannabis use on anxiety and on the efficacy of benzodiazepines. In some patients, the benzodiazepine dose can be gradually tapered and/or discontinued.

Degenerative Disc Disease and Associated Back Pain and Spasm

Ms. Smith is a 50-year-old hotel maid with a long history of significant low back pain made worse by her work duties. She has been followed by you for several years and has worsening degenerative disc disease and associated back pain and spasm. Her symptoms are no longer responding to NSAIDs and local analgesic creams. Also, she is experiencing recurrent heartburn from use of NSAIDs. She states that the back pain is "killing her" and wants to know if she should start taking opioids or even "marijuana." What advice should you give her?

Response: Chronic pain is the most common symptom for which medical cannabis is used. It is not uncommon for the progression of degenerative disc disease to necessitate increasingly potent pain relievers for the patient to maintain function. You should tell Ms. Smith that currently there are few good scientific studies of the pain-relieving effects of cannabis. There is, however, a large body of anecdotal cases suggesting that cannabis can be safely used for mild to moderate myofascial, neuropathic, or arthritic pain and cannabis can be used to mitigate the need for higher or more frequent doses of opioids. You can tell Ms. Smith that opioids are best not used for chronic non-malignant pain, and much safer, less addictive alternative medications need to be tried first.

You could explain that while psychological or, rarely, physical dependence on cannabis is possible, it is generally not a serious condition and can be managed much more simply and quickly, than opioid dependence.

Anxiety and Insomnia

After chronic pain, anxiety and insomnia are the next most frequent symptoms for which patients will ask their primary care provider for medical cannabis. Throughout recorded history, there has been anecdotal evidence of cannabis helping to relieve anxiety, perceived stress, and sleep problems.

Conversely, a small percentage of persons who use higher doses of cannabis recreationally commonly complain of acute onset of anxiety and paranoia. This is especially true of the higher potency cannabis used for recreational purposes. Studies of recreational users of cannabis suggest that they tend to use cannabis to self-medicate their pre-existing anxiety. In addition, it has been reported that people with symptoms of psychosis are more likely to use cannabis recreationally. It is not clear if there is any causal connection, but it appears likely that people use cannabis to mitigate their pre-existing symptoms.

Anxiety is multifaceted. It can manifest in several ways, including panic disorder, social anxiety disorder (SAD), and/or generalized anxiety disorder (GAD). THC is commonly felt to be an anxiolytic in most persons; however, CBD may also have a significant impact on anxiety, especially in SAD. Its anxiolytic effects are due to decreased activity in the limbic system.[59]

Recent studies show that CBD decreases fatty acid amide hydrolase (FAAH), the enzyme that breaks down anandamide, one of the two endogenous endocannabinoid neurotransmitters. It is postulated that an increase in naturally occurring anandamide can have significant anxiolytic effects, without the psychomotor effects of THC.[56]

A 2014 Vanderbilt University study[57] found CB1 receptors in the central nucleus of the amygdala in a mouse model. The amygdala is the part of the brain involved in emotional responses to pain and in the autonomic components of emotion such as heart rate, blood pressure, respiration, and conscious perception of emotions. The researchers theorized that the natural endocannabinoid system regulates anxiety and the response to stress by decreasing the excitatory signals. They also suggested that acute, severe emotional stress or chronic stress causes a reduction in the endocannabinoids and that without their buffering, anxiety increases.

The paradox is that the exogenous cannabinoids from cannabis may initially reduce anxiety, but with chronic use the receptors become down-regulated and anxiety increases. It is postulated that this can create a cycle leading to increasing doses and frequency of cannabis use and possible addiction or dependence syndromes.

The Vanderbilt University study shows that increasing AEA, one of the endocannabinoids, can effectively treat anxiety. It is felt that both THC and CBD impact anxiety in the ECS: THC by stimulating the same CB1 receptors as AEA, and CBD by indirectly increasing the levels of AEA at the receptors.

A Brazilian study in the *Journal of Psychopharmacology*[59] showed that CBD can be safely used to treat social anxiety disorder (SAD), which occurs in up to 12 percent of the population. This small study, using sophisticated cerebral blood flow imaging studies, showed CBD modulates activity in the limbic and paralimbic areas of the brain, significantly decreasing subjective anxiety.

CBD AND ANXIETY

Perceived stress is a major risk factor for the development of depression and anxiety. Using CBD to inhibit the AEA-degrading enzyme FAAH has been shown to reverse stress-induced anxiety in a mouse model. It did not affect anxiety in non-stressed mice. Additionally, central AEA levels could predict stress-induced anxiety behaviors.[58]

CBD has been shown in higher-quality studies to have anxiolytic effects in anxiety-prone and normal individuals. Several animal and human studies have shown that CBD alone can have measurable anxiolytic effects. CBD has been shown to be superior to placebo in reducing anxiety in patients with both generalized and social anxiety disorder.[59,60]

| *Not recommended for panic disorder.*

Panic disorder is a serious condition marked by recurrent episodes of severe anxiety. It occurs in about 1.25 percent of the population. It usually starts in the teens or early twenties, the same time that young adults start to experiment with recreational cannabis. There is evidence of a genetic predisposition to panic disorder. It usually occurs in response to a major life event or stressful period of time. After onset of panic attacks, the patient may start experiencing chronic anticipatory anxiety because of the fear of another attack.

A recent large population-based study[61] showed that lifetime cannabis use was significantly associated with increased risk of lifetime panic attack history after adjusting for sociodemographic variables. It was also significantly associated with past-year panic attacks. Earlier studies have shown similar findings. Persons dependent on cannabis appear to be most at risk for panic episodes. Persons with pre-existing panic disorder can have a worsening of their anxiety from cannabis use, and it is therefore not recommended in this patient population.

POST-TRAUMATIC STRESS DISORDER

Post-traumatic stress disorder (PTSD) may develop in a small percentage of persons exposed to emotionally traumatic events or threats. It is marked by hyperarousal, recurring flashbacks, irritability, outbursts of anger, and avoidance behaviors. There has been a marked increase in the number of persons diagnosed with PTSD with the return of Afghanistan and Iraqi war veterans. The Veterans Administration estimates that 11–20 percent of returning veterans have the disorder. There are no good pharmaceutical agents for the treatment of PTSD. Patients often end up on a cocktail of potent "off-label" drugs but still have poor symptom control.

PTSD is classified as an anxiety disorder in the DSM-IV manual. Twin studies have shown some evidence of a hereditary susceptibility. Alcohol and drug abuse often occur concomitantly, confusing the clinical picture. A large population-based cross-sectional study[62] showed that lifetime diagnosis of PTSD was significantly associated with lifetime and current cannabis use. The studies' researchers suggested a putative causal association between the onset of PTSD and cannabis use.

Research has consistently demonstrated that the ECS plays a significant role in PTSD. People with PTSD have significantly increased CB1 receptor levels, compared to healthy controls.[63,64] Because of this, individuals with PTSD may have a short-term reduction in PTSD symptoms, especially hyperarousal symptoms, with the use of cannabis.[65] However, longer-term use may lead to tolerance and increased difficulty with cannabis dependence symptoms.[66] There are anecdotal observations of the efficacy of cannabis for PTSD symptoms, but no good research at this time.

A large observational study of 2,276 Veterans Administration PTSD patients,[67] showed that those who never used cannabis had significantly lower symptom severity than those who started or continued to use cannabis. Also, cannabis users who stopped using it had significantly lower levels of PTSD symptoms at follow-up. In general, use of cannabis was associated with worsening of PTSD symptoms. The study showed a dose-response effect, with more cannabis use being associated with worse PTSD symptoms. However, because of the design of the study, it could not be determined if patients who used cannabis had worse PTSD symptoms than those who did not use it.

Dr. Suzanne Sisley has been treating veterans with PTSD for over 20 years. She has been trying to conduct serious research on this topic for many years. In 2009, she originally designed a study entitled *Placebo-Controlled, Triple-Blind, Randomized Crossover Pilot Study of the Safety and Efficacy of Five Different Potencies of Smoked or Vaporized Marijuana in 76 Veterans with Chronic, Treatment-Resistant Post-traumatic Stress Disorder (PTSD)*. The intent of the study is to test several cultivars of cannabis with different CBD:THC ratios and potencies. However, due to serious inefficiencies at the National Institute of Drug Abuse (NIDA) and the inability of the University of Mississippi cannabis program to create the correct cultivars of cannabis, this study has yet to go forward.

Despite a number of states approving PTSD as a qualifying medical condition for medical cannabis, there is no evidence to support its use for treatment of PTSD. Other data suggest that while THC may aggravate PTSD symptoms, use of CBD alone may be useful for treating PTSD symptoms.[68]

PSYCHOSIS/SCHIZOPHRENIA

Psychosis, or schizophrenia, is manifested by delusions, hallucinations, paranoia, and disorganized thinking, speech, and concentration. About 3 percent of people experience a psychotic episode in their life time. Often, alcohol use or drugs are the major contributing cause of a psychotic episode. The onset of schizophrenia is usually in the late teens or early twenties, the same time that most young people begin to experiment with recreational cannabis. This makes it difficult to draw conclusions from the available scant data.

Consumption of cannabis can induce a temporary psychosis, with symptoms of disorganized thoughts, paranoia, and hallucinations. These symptoms are seen in many psychiatric conditions, not just schizophrenia. However, temporary psychosis is usually due to rapid and excessive intake of THC, which is most common in recreational cannabis users. Of concern is the development of long-term psychosis or other mental illness as a result of cannabis use.

At this time, the available body of scientific evidence cannot provide a definitive answer as to whether cannabis use causes psychosis/schizophrenia or triggers a latent condition in some cases. The risk of causing psychosis should be seriously considered prior to initiating cannabis therapeutically. A prior psychiatric history consistent with psychosis or a strong family history of schizophrenia should be considered a contraindication to the use of cannabis.

Several studies have shown the concomitant presence of CBD can mitigate THC-induced psychosis.[13–16] In clinical trials, CBD has been shown to result in similar reduction in psychotic symptoms in schizophrenic patients, compared to antipsychotic medications, but with much fewer side effects.[69,70] In a case report of a patient with schizophrenia who could not tolerate antipsychotic medications, a significant reduction in psychotic symptoms was reported with use of high-dose CBD for four weeks, with the return of symptoms after discontinuation of the CBD.[71] Further large-scale studies are planned to determine if CBD is an effective alternative treatment for schizophrenic patients.[72]

INSOMNIA

The term *insomnia* refers to difficulty falling asleep, known as *onset insomnia*, and difficulty staying asleep or early-morning awakening. Insomnia of some sort occurs in up to 30 percent of the population during their lifetime, with a point prevalence of about 10 percent of the population. The ECS has been shown to have a regulatory effect on sleep. Both THC and 11-OH-THC, the metabolite from orally ingested cannabis, have been shown to decrease the time to fall asleep, which is known as *sleep latency*. Lower doses of THC, approximately 20 mg, are superior to higher doses and can reduce sleep latency by an hour. THC also increases the duration of sleep. Higher doses are not as effective due to the psychoactive effects of THC. Lower doses are associated with less of a "hangover" effect in the morning.

A 2010 study[74] has shown THC to be superior to amitriptyline for sleep quality in patients with fibromyalgia. There is also suggestive evidence of a beneficial central effect on sleep apnea.

CBD has mixed effects on sleep. At low doses, CBD has been shown to provoke wakefulness and, at higher doses, to increase sedation and sleep time.[75-77] CBD, in combination with THC, appears to counteract the sleep-inducing effects of THC and to improve awareness. Therefore, low percentage CBD with higher percentage THC cannabis should be used for treatment of insomnia.

Tolerance may develop to these positive insomnia effects of THC with chronic high-dose use. In addition, persons withdrawing from THC can sometimes develop adverse sleep effects.

An older (1981) study of 15 patients[75] has shown positive effects on insomnia with 160 mg doses of CBD, alone. However, the findings of this study are not consistent with those of newer studies.

Benzodiazepines, the current first-line drugs for insomnia, convert deep sleep to lighter sleep, with a modest increase in the duration of the sleep but a decrease in the quality. They are also much more habituating than cannabis.

TREATMENT RECOMMENDATIONS

There are many FDA-approved and generally recognized medications for both insomnia and anxiety. Long-term use of most of the traditional agents is not recommended, and there are real risks of dependency and accidental overdose, especially with the potent benzodiazepines.

If appropriate, the clinician can safely recommend the use of cannabinoids for treatment of the symptoms of anxiety and insomnia in carefully selected patients. Based on the discussion above, the clinician should take a thorough medical and psychiatric history to identify risk factors for psychiatric side-effects from the use of cannabis, including worsening of anxiety or psychosis. In addition, since onset of anxiety and panic attacks may be associated with cannabis dependence or addiction syndromes, prior cannabis, alcohol, or drug dependence or a family history of these should be evaluated prior to initiating medical cannabis.

The prior use of cannabis recreationally or medically without side-effects is always a good indicator of future effects. The cannabis dose, as always, should be started out low and titrated up slowly. Again, the literature suggests that higher and faster dosing of THC are associated with onset of anxiety. Also, chronic use can gradually lead to secondary anxiety for reasons previously discussed.

CBD, alone, is recommended for the treatment of anxiety. As discussed in an earlier chapter, CBD oil derived from industrial hemp seed and stalks is legal and available over-the-counter in many states. The oil is very safe and can be ingested or vaporized. If a cannabis containing THC is used, it should be one with a low percentage of THC and high percentage of CBD.

For treatment of chronic anxiety, an edible product may be preferred for its long duration of the therapeutic effect. However, the patient will need to experiment with the wide array of edibles that are available. The effects, potency, and onset and duration of action of even the same brand of edible may vary due to quality-control issues with most local or regional brands of cannabis edibles.

For treatment of episodic anxiety, vaporized or smoked cannabis may be preferable due to the patient's ability to gradually titrate the dose for symptom control over a short period of time.

For the treatment of chronic insomnia, many patients prefer to ingest an edible about an hour or more before bedtime. THC provides all of the somnolent effects. The onset of action with ingested cannabis is slower, and the duration of effect is much longer. However, a too-high dose of THC can cause annoying psychoactive effects, hindering sleep onset.

For episodic insomnia, vaporized or smoked cannabis can lead to the rapid onset of somnolence in about 15 minutes, although the effect is short lived, about 45–60 minutes.

A low-CBD and high-THC cannabis product is recommended for treatment of insomnia.

Anxiety- and Pain-Related Insomnia

One of your patients requests medical cannabis for her insomnia. She has not had a good outcome from the use of several different hypnotic medications. Upon further questioning, you discover she has onset insomnia, associated with anxiety and ruminating before falling asleep as well as early-morning wakening due to neck and back pain from arthritis. What cannabis regimen would you recommend?

Response: This is an excellent example of the kind of patient that should do well with cannabis therapy. She has failed trials of traditional hypnotic medications, and she has both onset insomnia from anxiety and early-morning wakening for arthritic pain. She would benefit from a long-acting dose of cannabis that would last through the night. Cannabis with an equal ratio of THC to CBD might be tried initially for the pain- and anxiety-relieving effects of THC and the muscle-relaxing and anti-inflammatory effects of CBD.

The best vehicles for delivery of the cannabis would be a cannabis edible or beverage plus a slow-release cannabis patch. The cannabinoids in the ingested cannabis will be subject to the liver's first-pass effect, resulting in the maximum therapeutic effects occurring in 1–2 hours but lasting around 6 hours. The patient should be advised to take the edible 1 hour before bedtime and to apply the patch 30 minutes before bedtime.

She will need to experiment with the edibles and patches to determine the correct dose. Patches can be cut to vary the dose. As with all cannabinoid medications, advise the patient to start low and titrate up slowly.

INFLAMMATION AND SPASTICITY

Although patients do not often come to a clinician asking for cannabis specifically for inflammation or spasm, these two symptoms are often part and parcel of chronic pain syndrome. However, cannabinoids have an entirely different mechanism of action on these symptoms from that of pain.

CBD'S EFFECTS ON INFLAMMATION

Cannabinoids work in a variety of ways to reduce inflammation. While it has been repeatedly shown that cannabinoids, especially CBD, are associated with anti-inflammatory properties, there is likely more than one mode of action. Cannabis has anti-inflammatory effects in the CNS via CB2 receptors found on microglial cells. In the periphery, CB2 receptors are found on immune cells such as monocytes, macrophages, B cells, and T cells. They are also known to be on mast cells, which are components of the inflammatory response system.[78]

CB2 receptors are also found throughout the spleen, thymus gland, and tonsils. In the gastrointestinal tract, CB2 receptors are believed to modulate the intestinal inflammatory response that causes Crohn's disease and ulcerative colitis.[78,86]

It has been shown that cannabinoids work through the ECS to reduce or prevent inflammation. Specifically, CBD indirectly activates CB2 receptors on immune system cells. This action is implicated in a variety of modulating functions. CB2 activation results in a reduction in the release of cytokines and chemokines, both pro-inflammatory substances. This also induces apoptosis, programmed cell death. The immune system cells are also involved: CB2 activation inhibits T-cell receptor signaling and increases retention of marginal zone B cells.[78] Clinical trials have shown that CBD can be moderately effective in reducing inflammation in multiple sclerosis,[79] traumatic brain injury,[80] inflammatory bowel disease,[81] Alzheimer's disease,[82] and rheumatoid arthritis.[83]

A recent study of a viral model of multiple sclerosis,[79] showed that CBD decreased transmigration of blood leukocytes and cytokines in the brain and attenuated the activation of microglia in the CNS. These effects were long lasting. The investigators believe that their findings demonstrate that CBD has a "significant therapeutic potential" for the treatment of pathologies with an inflammatory component.

A population-based cross-sectional study of cannabis users, compared to non-users, showed that recent users of cannabis had significantly lower levels of C-reactive protein, a marker of inflammation, than those who had never used cannabis.[84] However, the etiology of this is poorly understood.

BETA-CARYOPHYLLENE'S EFFECTS ON INFLAMMATION

Beta-caryophyllene (BCP) is another substance believed to have anti-inflammatory effects when present in high amounts (4–37 percent) in cannabis oil. Since BCP is a terpenophenolic constituent of cannabis plants, it is a phytocannabinoid. Caryophyllene oxide is the component that is used to train drug-sniffing dogs how to identify cannabis.

BCP is a selective agonist of peripheral CB2 receptors. It has no binding affinity to CB1 receptors. In addition to being present in cannabis, BCP is found in high amounts in many plants and spices. It has been shown to avert inflammation and decrease neuropathic pain in a mouse model.[85] It is present in clove oil, black pepper, hops, basil, and many flowers. It is an FDA-approved food additive. Currently, there are no high-quality clinical studies in humans.

THC'S EFFECTS ON INFLAMMATION

While many of the anti-inflammatory effects of cannabis can be attributed to the non-psychoactive cannabinoid CBD, THC may have a role to play as well. CB1 receptors have been found on immune system cells. Recent studies show that administration of THC into mice triggered marked apoptosis in T cells and dendritic cells, resulting in immunosuppression. In addition, other studies showed that cannabinoids downregulate cytokine and chemokine production and, in some models, upregulate T-regulatory cells as a mechanism to suppress inflammatory responses.[78]

As with the other clinical effects of cannabinoids, much clinical research on the anti-inflammatory effects of CBD and to a lesser extent, THC, needs to be conducted.

EFFECTS OF CANNABIS COMPARED TO NSAIDS

There are many FDA-approved, generally recognized anti-inflammatory medications available at this time. None of the effects of these have been seriously compared to cannabinoids in high-quality studies. Cannabis may be considered as an adjuvant therapy in carefully selected patients who are already taking NSAIDs. A 1:1 ratio of THC:CBD is recommended. The combined analgesic, anti-inflammatory, anti-spasticity effects, as well as possible beneficial mood effects, may make this a useful adjunct therapy.

EFFECTS ON SPASTICITY

Cannabis has long been postulated to reduce muscle spasm and spasticity. This has been based mostly on anecdotal observations. Dr. William O'Shaughnessy reported in 1842 that cannabis effectively controlled spasticity in cases of tetanus. Small studies from the 1970s suggested that cannabis controlled muscle spasms in patients with spinal cord injuries. However, the fact that THC and CBD can reduce myofascial and neuropathic pain is a confounding factor in determining how much relief of spasm and spasticity is actually taking place.

EFFECTS ON SPINAL CORD INJURY

Individuals with spinal cord injury often develop chronic spasticity from injury to upper motor neurons in the CNS. This presents as an increase in tonic stretch reflexes (muscle tone), with exaggerated tendon jerks resulting from hyperexcitability of the stretch reflex. This spasticity affects the person's quality of life (QOL) and activities of daily living (ADL). The available medications and therapy are usually only partially effective and are associated with significant side-effects. Anecdotal case reports support that cannabis has a relaxing effect on the spastic muscle, perhaps through the inhibition of polysynaptic reflexes.[87]

EFFECTS ON MULTIPLE SCLEROSIS

Most of the studies of the use of cannabis for spasticity are reports of its efficacy in treating patients with multiple sclerosis (MS). MS is the most common debilitating neurologic disease of younger persons. It is a chronic condition marked by spasticity, pain, and tremor as primary symptoms. It is the most studied neurologic condition for cannabis therapy. However, there is only limited evidence of cannabis's effects, many of them case reports. Anecdotally, MS patients have reported subjective relief of spasm and pain, minutes after smoking cannabis. Other anecdotal observations include a profound effect on spasm, tremors, bladder control, speech, and eyesight.[88] However, there were issues with worsening of balance control.[89]

A survey of MS patients in 2002 showed that half of MS patients were regularly using cannabis to control their spasms.[90]

A 2008 University of San Diego study[91] showed that inhaled cannabis significantly reduced objective measures of pain intensity and spasticity in patients with MS in a placebo-controlled, randomized clinical trial. They concluded that "smoked cannabis was superior to placebo in reducing spasticity and pain in patients with multiple sclerosis and provided some benefit beyond currently prescribed treatment."

In mouse models of viral-induced demyelinating disease, cannabinoids have been shown to lessen MS symptoms and halt progression of the disease.[92]

A well-designed but small, short-term study of smoked cannabis[79] showed that it was superior to placebo in reducing spasticity and pain in MS patients. However, there were also significant adverse cognitive effects.

The current National Multiple Sclerosis Society recommendation on the use of cannabis suggests that it can have negative cognitive effects. This is important information because MS patients may already have cognitive impairment from the disease. The society did note that a recent clinical trial of Sativex significantly improved spasticity and resulted in some pain relief in some MS patients. Additional clinical research was recommended.

(*See* www.nationalmssociety.org/Treating-MS/Complementary-Alternative-Medicines/Marijuana.)

None of the available evidence provides a good clinical understanding of cannabinoids' anti-spasticity effects at a cellular or molecular level.

TREATMENT RECOMMENDATION

There are several effective and generally recognized medications for spasticity, and none of these have been compared in a study with cannabinoids. The potential cognitive side-effects of cannabis in MS patients and spinal cord injury patients, who may have associated cognitive deficits, are a real concern, and cannabis is not a recommended therapy for MS or persons with pre-existing cognitive deficits, at this time.

APPETITE STIMULATION

Although CBD does not have any effect on the appetite, there are plenty of anecdotal, and often humorous, observations about the appetite-stimulating effects of THC. Indeed, cannabis has been shown to increase food intake and body weight in healthy subjects. A decades-old study of recreational cannabis users showed that smoking cannabis increased calorie intake by 40 percent.[93] However, a more recent large population-based study showed that long-term regular cannabis smokers are actually slimmer than matched non-smokers. They found rates of obesity about one-third less in persons who smoke cannabis at least three times a week. This may be due to increased metabolism from the effects of the cannabinoids. However, there were several significant confounding effects in the study design.[95]

It is believed that the ECS may serve as a regulator of feeding behavior and reward behavior. The ECS has been shown to be intimately involved with the pleasure that people receive from eating food, known as the *hedonic effect*. There is also research to suggest that CB1 receptors in the hypothalamus are involved in the reward and motivational aspects of eating.

Numerous disease states and conditions, such as cancer, HIV, and the adverse effects of chemotherapy, can result in markedly reduced appetite and cachexia. This significantly impacts the body's ability to heal. THC has been shown to have appetite-stimulating effects by signaling food craving within the brain. Studies of AIDS patients have shown that low doses of pure oral THC analogue can double the appetite, as measured by a visual analogue scale.

Like antiemetic effects, most of the high-quality studies regarding appetite stimulation were done with the synthetic THC analogues Marinol and Cesamet. Again, the results of studies of these pharmaceuticals are not felt to be generalizable to cannabis, due to the entourage effect of CBD, other cannabinoids, and terpenes. These older studies suggest sustained improvement in appetite and modest weight gain, especially at higher doses. However, the adverse effects limit the utility of these two pharmaceuticals.

USE IN AIDS AND CANCER PATIENTS

Two small placebo-controlled studies of the use of cannabis for AIDS patients confirmed a beneficial effect on food intake and body weight.[95,96] Studies of AIDS patients show improved body weight and mood and decreased nausea. Sustained efficacy of cannabis's appetite-stimulating effects has been shown for at least seven months. The stimulation of appetite from one dose can last 24 hours or longer.

There are currently no high-quality studies on the benefit of cannabis, ingested or smoked, for cancer-related anorexia or cachexia.

In recent years, Megestrol has been shown to be superior to cannabis for weight gain in cancer and AIDS patients. Cannabis is therefore not recommended for isolated stimulation of appetite. However, cannabis may be an excellent adjunct medication for cancer or HIV patients who have a combination of pain, anxiety, nausea, and anorexia.

USE FOR EATING DISORDERS

Eating disorders affect millions of Americans, mostly girls and young women. Eating disorders have the highest mortality rate of any mental illness. Eating disorders such as anorexia nervosa and bulimia are thought to develop as an exaggerated response to cultural standards of beauty. In addition, the effects of food deprivation are thought to provide the patient with some sense of control over their bodies.

A small study of women with eating disorders, using positron emission tomography (PET) scanning, showed that the insula, the part of the brain responsible for integrating the taste of food with our emotional reward response to eating, was significantly underactive in these women. It is noted that persons with eating disorders are not without hunger.

A recent high-quality study of 24 women with severe long-lasting anorexia nervosa showed that synthetic THC pills resulted in around 2 pounds more weight gain over four weeks than placebo. Another small study found no significant effect of THC on weight gain, but THC had several psychological adverse effects.[97] The researchers concluded that longer treatment might achieve benefits, but larger study sample sizes were needed.

TREATMENT RECOMMENDATION

Because eating disorders are fundamentally psychological disorders, and patients with eating disorders already have intact hunger sensation, cannabis is not indicated nor has it been shown to be effective.

Eating Disorder in an 18-Year-Old Female

A father brings his 18-year-old daughter to the clinic to discuss her eating disorder. He is frustrated with her worsening condition. He asks you to start her on medical cannabis to gain weight. What can you tell him?

Response: After ensuring that the adult daughter wants her father to be involved with her care, you can discuss exactly what treatment she has already had. Then you can tell them that although THC is a potentially effective appetite stimulant for wasting disorders, including HIV, it has not been shown to be effective for other forms of cachexia such as eating disorders. Patients with eating disorders have intact hunger sensation, and regular cannabis users tend to be slimmer than their counterparts.

In addition, any medication used as part of her recovery would need to be supervised by a clinician who is managing her entire treatment plan, usually a psychiatrist.

Nausea and Vomiting

CHEMOTHERAPY-INDUCED NAUSEA AND VOMITING

Cannabis has long been associated with alleviating nausea and vomiting in cancer patients undergoing chemotherapy. This condition is known as *chemotherapy-induced nausea and vomiting (CINV)*.

Numerous *in vitro* and *in vivo* studies suggest that the ECS is involved in many functions of the gastrointestinal system, including fibrogenesis, inflammation, motility, and nausea and vomiting.

Most of the high-quality studies were done with the synthetic THC analogues Marinol and Cesamet. These studies are not generally transferable to cannabis-related medication.[98,99] These two drugs were studied for prevention of CINV. The results showed some clinical benefit for CINV, but these results are inferior to those of the more recent 5-HT3 antagonists and NK1 antagonist pharmaceuticals. However, these synthetic THC analogues had a much worse adverse-effect profile than cannabis. There are actually no placebo-controlled human studies of the antiemetic efficacy of cannabis. However, anecdotally, most cancer patients prefer smoked cannabis for CINV. This could be due to its concomitant mood elevation effects.

Since the 1990s and the introduction of serotonin receptor antagonists (5-HT3), there are now several effective and safe FDA-approved medications for the treatment of CINV and episodic nausea and vomiting.

TREATMENT RECOMMENDATION

Because of the available superior and safe medications, and the adverse psychoactive effects of the THC, monotherapy use of synthetic THC or cannabis for isolated nausea and vomiting is not recommended.

However, cannabis can have a wide variety of symptom-modifying effects in cancer and AIDS patients, including pain relief, anti-anxiety effects, and improved appetite and mood, in addition to the rapid onset of anti-nausea effects. Therefore, cannabis may be a good adjunct therapy for carefully selected cancer and AIDS patients with a wide array of these symptoms.

CANNABINOID HYPEREMESIS SYNDROME

Cannabinoid hyperemesis syndrome, marked by recurrent nausea, vomiting and abdominal colicky pain, was first described in 2004.[27] It is rare and occurs only after years of regular use of cannabinoids. The gastrointestinal symptoms are usually severe and cyclical over months. A hallmark of this condition is that the nausea and vomiting resolve after discontinuing the cannabinoids. Other diagnoses should be ruled out.

The pathogenic mechanism of this condition is not known. Cannabinoid toxicity or functional effects of chronic cannabinoids on the hypothalamus have been postulated.

Chemotherapy-Induced Nausea and Vomiting

A patient with CINV is not responding well to all of the available antiemetic drugs. He does not want to use cannabis because he thinks it is an addictive drug. What can you tell him to encourage him to try cannabis for its adjuvant antiemetic effects?

Response: You can tell the patient that cannabis is an effective adjuvant to the currently available medications. The prescription pill form of the medication tends to have more unpleasant side-effects, such as anxiety and psychoactive effects, compared to more easily titrated cannabis. Cannabis also contains CBD and other terpenes that enhance the therapeutic effects of the THC.

Although approximately 10 percent of people who use cannabis can become psychologically, or rarely, physically dependent on cannabis, you are going to start him on the lowest effective dose and monitor for the possible occurrence of dependence. Withdrawal from THC dependence is almost always mild and short term.

Finally, you can tell him that cannabis can have several other positive clinical effects on cancer-associated symptoms, such as reducing anxiety and pain and increasing appetite.

Cancer and Tumors

For more than two decades, cannabinoids, especially THC, have been known to have antitumor effects. More recent basic scientific studies have shown that several other cannabinoids, including CBD, have similarly potent antitumor effects.

This antitumor effect appears to work on benign and malignant tumors and has been shown to be effective in *in vitro* and *in vivo* for a variety of rodent tumors.[100–102] It is postulated that cannabinoids cause antitumor effects by various mechanisms, including the induction of cell death through apoptosis, inhibition of cell growth, and inhibition of tumor angiogenesis invasion and metastasis.[100–102]

Cannabinoids induce apoptosis in transformed cells but do not affect normal cells. Apoptosis is a form of tightly regulated programmed cell death. The studies suggest that cannabinoids, via the CB1 receptors, also protect normal cells. These antitumor and cytoprotective effects of various cannabinoids have been shown in a variety of animal model tumors. Another hypothesis for antitumor effects may be due to the anti-inflammatory effects on tumors such as colon cancer.[103] Chronic inflammation has been shown to be a causal factor in an increasing number of cancers.

PROSTATE CANCER

Experimental murine models have shown that cannabinoids can have a depressant effect on the male reproductive system, decreasing circulating testosterone and spermatogenesis.[104]

Prostate cancer is the most common form of cancer in American men. Available evidence shows that prostate tissue possesses cannabinoid receptors and that these receptors cause an anti-androgenic effect. A 2012 review[105] of all of the available basic science evidence of the role of cannabinoids in prostate cancer revealed that prostate cancer cells possess increased expression of both CB1 and CB2 receptors, compared to normal prostate cells. Stimulation of these receptors with cannabinoid agonists resulted in a decrease in cell viability, increased apoptosis, and decreased androgen-receptor protein expression and prostate-specific antigen (PSA) excretion.

The available research suggests that cannabinoids should be further evaluated for the management of prostate cancer with *in vivo* and clinical trials.

MELANOMA

Melanoma comprises only 2 percent of skin cancer cases, but it is the most serious type of skin cancer. In the United States, there are more than 76,000 new cases and almost 10,000 deaths annually. Melanoma is caused by overproliferation of abnormal melanocytes. Its incidence is increasing exponentially, especially in younger age groups, probably due to sun and tanning-booth exposure.

Cells perform a process known as *autophagy* that cleans out intracellular debris. This is done with the help of lysosomes that contain enzymes to break down the organelles and proteins. Initially, autophagy is helpful in preventing cancer; however, the same process can be used by cancer cells to help maintain their survival. Also, autophagy can result in apoptosis, programmed cell death.

A very recent *in vitro* and *in vivo* study[106] showed that THC alone, and THC combined with CBD, increased autophagy-dependent apoptosis in melanoma in a dose-dependent manner. The effect was enhanced by CBD in combination with THC. In addition, normal cells were protected from the process. This treatment worked better than the currently available alkylating agents, with many fewer side effects. The cannabis medication worked on both BRAF-mutated and BRAF-wildtype. The investigators noted that the molecular mechanisms connecting autophagy to apoptosis are poorly understood.[106]

HEPATOCELLULAR CANCER

Hepatocellular cancer (HCC) is a significant cause of death in the United States. When HCC progresses to advanced stages, there are few treatment options. An *in vitro* study[107] of THC showed that it reduced the viability of HCC cell lines through stimulation of CB2 receptors and the initiation of autophagy. Further study was recommended by the researchers.

BREAST CANCER

Breast cancer is a significant cause of morbidity and mortality in women in developed countries. An *in vitro* study[108] of breast cancer cell lines found that CBD induced apoptosis, independent of the CB1, CB2, or vanilloid receptors. CBD inhibited the survival of both estrogen-positive and estrogen-negative cell lines, with a concentration-dependent effect. There was little effect on normal mammary cells. Other studies have also shown the antitumor effect of cannabinoids in preclinical models of breast cancer.[110,111]

COLON CANCER
This is the third most common form of cancer in adults in the United States. Studies using murine models have demonstrated an antitumor effect when CBD was administered together with a known cancer-causing agent.[112] The effect of the protection appeared to be mediated through CB1 receptors.[113]

LUNG CANCER
Lung cancer is the most common cancer in adults in developed countries. There is *in vivo* evidence that CBD plays a role in the expression of intercellular adhesion molecule-1 (ICAM-1). In lung cancer, it was shown to upregulate ICAM-1, which resulted in decreased metastasis and invasiveness.[114] THC was also shown to have antiangiogenic and antiproliferative effects.

GLIOBLASTOMA MULTIFORME AND GLIOMA
Glioblastoma multiforme and glioma are both highly treatment-resistant brain cancers. CBD has been shown to induce apoptosis in glioma cell lines and to induce regression of glioma tumors in murine models, while it protects normal glial cells of astroglial and oligodendroglial lineages from apoptosis mediated by CB1.[101]

A synthetic version of CBD has recently been granted an orphan-drug designation by the FDA for treatment of these malignancies.

Neurologic Conditions
The American Academy of Neurology conducted a review of research done from 1948 until 2013 to determine the efficacy and safety of medical cannabis for multiple sclerosis (MS), epilepsy, and movement disorders. The review included 34 studies, of which 8 were determined to be high quality. The authors concluded that cannabis extract, THC, and Sativex are probably effective in reducing centrally-mediated pain, painful spasms, and spasticity-related pain. It was found that Sativex is probably effective for reducing the number of bladder voids per day, but

THC and cannabis extracts are probably ineffective for over-active bladder. Cannabis probably has no effect on tremors: it was ineffective for levodopa-induced dyskinesias in patients with Parkinson's disease. The authors could not draw any firm conclusions regarding the efficacy of medical cannabis for Huntington's disease, Tourette syndrome, cervical dystonia, or epilepsy.

EPILEPSY

Epilepsy is one of the most common neurologic disorders in children. There are approximately 466,000 pediatric patients in the United States. Up to 20 percent of these cases are pharma-coresistant to currently available treatments and are deemed "medically intractable." Furthermore, it is recognized that many of those whose medication does provide relief suffer side-effects that are severe enough for an alternative to be sought.

One recent study consisted of surveying parents of children using non-standardized CBD-enriched cannabis preparations for intractable epilepsy. Of the 19 children in the survey, 13 had Dravet syndrome, 4 had Doose syndrome, 1 had Lennox-Gastaut syndrome, and 1 had idiopathic epilepsy. The average number of antiepileptic drugs tried before using CBD was 12.84 percent. Parents of children who tried CBD reported a reduction in their children's seizure frequency. Of these, 11 percent reported complete remissions of seizures for at least a month, 42 percent reported a greater than 80 percent reduction in seizure frequency, and 32 percent reported a 25–60 percent reduction. The side-effects of CBD were generally mild.[117]

In the past decade, many other anecdotal observations and case studies by doctors and parents have been reported.

There is sufficient research on epilepsy and CBD to show a beneficial clinical effect. Several early studies confirmed reduced seizure frequency with use of CBD.[5,115] There are few, if any, safety concerns with CBD use, and the available evidence supports the use of CBD for treatment-resistant epilepsy in adults.[116] The use of CBD for treatment-resistant pediatric epilepsies, such as Dravet syndrome and Lennox-Gastaut syndrome, is also supported.[117] A phase III clinical trial study of CBD for Dravet syndrome is promising.[118] Other studies are planned.

PARKINSON'S DISEASE

There are several studies on the use of CBD for Parkinson's disease. CBD has been shown to reduce general and motor symptoms and to heighten the patient's sense of well-being and improve quality of life.[119] It reduced medication-associated dystonia by 20–50 percent.[120] It also reduced the frequency of rapid eye movement (REM) sleep disorder in Parkinson's patients.[121]

MULTIPLE SCLEROSIS

This was discussed in detail earlier in this chapter in the "Inflammation and Spasticity" section (*see* page 94).

Inflammatory Bowel Disease

Numerous *in vitro* and *in vivo* studies suggest that the endocannabinoid system (ECS) is involved in many functions of the gastrointestinal (GI) system, including inflammation, motility, and nausea and vomiting. However, most of the higher quality studies were done with synthetic THC analogues for prevention of CINV or for appetite stimulation.

Patients with Crohn's disease and ulcerative colitis, both forms of inflammatory bowel disease (IBD), anecdotally report significant beneficial effects of cannabis on nausea, appetite, and abdominal pain. There does not appear to be a beneficial effect on diarrhea.

CB2 receptors are found throughout the GI system, where they modulate the intestinal inflammatory response. Inflammation in the colon appears to increase CB2-receptor expression. This has been shown *in vitro* to be involved with inhibition of cytokine-related inflammation. Thus, the CB2 receptor is a potential therapeutic target for patients with IBD. Endocannabinoids play an important role in inhibiting unnecessary immune action upon the natural gut flora. Dysfunction of this system, perhaps from excess fatty acid amide hydrolase (FAAH) activity, could result in IBD. CB2 activation reduces gut motility in IBS patients and may also have a role in irritable bowel syndrome.

In the GI tract, CB1 receptors are expressed predominantly in the enteric nervous system, where they are thought to have an inhibitory effect on motility and secretory function through reduced acetylcholine release. CB1 receptors are also present to a lesser degree in the colonic epithelium and smooth muscle, where activation of the CB1 receptors may enhance epithelial healing.

A small randomized control study of smoked cannabis showed a significant response as measured by the Crohn's Disease Activity Index. However, the study evaluated only subjective improvement; there is no study showing objective evidence of improvement.[122]

Phase II studies of an oral cannabis-based pharmaceutical for ulcerative colitis are underway in Europe. The medication contains CBD:THC in a ratio of 20:1.

GLAUCOMA

Smoked marijuana was shown to lower intraocular pressure in some studies conducted in the 1970s and early 1980s. However, this effect lasted only about 4 hours. One expert reasoned that patients would have to use marijuana around the clock in order to effectively treat glaucoma. Standard medicines are generally more useful for people with glaucoma.

Addictions

Use of cannabis to help decrease opioid-seeking behaviors and to help discontinue medical use of opioids was discussed in the section of this chapter on pain (*see* page 81). However, recent studies suggest CBD may have a role in treating a wide array of addictions. Morgan and colleagues[123] found that the use of CBD by habitual tobacco smokers resulted in a 40 percent reduction in the number of cigarettes smoked, compared to no change in the control group given a placebo.

PART III

Medical Cannabis in Clinical Practice

CHAPTER 9

Overview

This chapter is designed to provide information on the distinct difference between prescribing medications in regular clinical practice and recommending cannabis for medical conditions. It focuses on the use of the THC and CBD cannabinoids as medicine. The chapter also briefly addresses recreational cannabis.

Previous chapters elucidated the mechanisms of action of the different endocannabinoids and the ECS. These chapters also explained that the endocannabinoids CBD and THC are present in high concentrations in the plant material and that they have been the most studied for their clinical application. There are dozens of other cannabinoids present in small amounts in cannabis, but although these are believed to have effects similar to THC or CBD, they have not been well studied.

As stated in Chapter 2, there are very few high-quality studies to support the use of medical cannabis for the variety of conditions for which it has been recommended.[1,2] Therefore, cannabis is never first-line treatment, and unless the laws change, clinicians cannot prescribe cannabis. Rather, they can recommend it if it is legal under current state law and deemed appropriate adjuvant therapy. (In the future there may be conditions—for example, anxiety, certain forms of epilepsy, chronic pain syndromes, and spasticity—for which cannabis becomes monotherapy.)

As discussed in Chapter 2, because cannabis is a Schedule I controlled substance at the federal level, it is against DEA and FDA regulations to prescribe it, even though it is legal to use for certain medical conditions in the state in which a clinician practices. The doctor can only *recommend* cannabis in a standard recommendation letter. An example of the official template letter for the State of California, Medical Marijuana Program, is included as Appendix B in this book. Chapter 11 gives guidance on writing recommendation letters for cannabis use.

Under current state and federal laws, cannabis cannot be prescribed by clinicians. Rather, they can recommend it by writing a letter of recommendation, which the patient then can obtain at a certified medical cannabis dispensary.

THC and CBD as Medicine

THC is the most well known and most medically active plant-based cannabinoid. As discussed in Chapter 2, the percent of THC in the plant material varies significantly, as does CBD. CBD is the next most studied cannabinoid. Low-THC and high-CBD cannabis has different indications, effects, and adverse reactions from high-THC, low-CBD cultivars and from cultivars with approximately equal proportions of THC and CBD. The following discussion highlights the differences.

The very low-THC and high-CBD cultivar (strain) of cannabis known as *Charlotte's Web* is legal in an increasing number of states for medical purposes. Many states that have not legalized cannabis with high THC levels have legalized Charlotte's Web and other cultivars with very low (0.3 percent) THC.

CBD, alone, acts through different pathways of the body than THC. It inhibits FAAH and results in higher levels of endocannabinoid neurotransmitters. It is most commonly used for certain rare pediatric seizure disorders, anxiety, nausea and vomiting, and inflammatory conditions.

Both THC and CBD are very safe when used appropriately, and there are relatively mild short-term side-effects from an excessive dose or accidental ingestion. However, when recommending cannabis therapy, the clinician must be cognizant of the possibility of the patient's developing cannabis dependence syndrome and associated psychosis. As discussed in later chapters, there are excellent screening tools to use prior to initiating cannabis therapy for evaluating the medication's efficacy and for monitoring the patient for the possible development of dependence syndrome during treatment.

Many studies of the safety of CBD have been done. It has been administered orally, by inhalation, and intravenously in several week-long to month-long trials as well as in acute, one-time doses. No neurologic, cardiac, psychiatric, or blood chemistry abnormalities have been identified.[5-10] Only some sedation was observed in patients who received high doses of CBD.[11]

Other than acute anxiety or transient psychosis in a minority of patients, the main side-effects of THC and its metabolite, 11-OH-THC, are psychoactive effects. In general, these tend to lessen over time and as the patient acquires more experience in titrating the medicine.

Both THC and CBD are very safe when used appropriately, and there are relatively mild short-term side-effects from an excessive dose or accidental ingestion. CBD, alone, is very safe.

Increased Psychoactive Effects

Your patient has been on medical cannabis for several years. He uses vaporized cannabis a few times a month for episodic spasms. He comes to you complaining of an increased amount of psychoactive effects from the same dose of vaporized cannabis. He has not changed his equipment, strain of cannabis, or use of other medications or alcohol. What advice can you give him?

Discussion: The psychoactive effects from cannabis are mediated by the THC component. Generally, after two weeks of use and practice in titrating the dose of cannabis, a patient has no psychoactive side-effects, or at least they are tolerable. A noticeable increase in the psychoactive effects is due to a higher amount of THC delivered to the CB1 receptors in the brain. Since the patient has not changed the cannabis dose or delivery system, the cannabis preparation he is now using must have a higher percentage of THC than that he was previously using.

There is very little in the way of standardization of THC content in cannabis dispensaries. The same strain name at the same dispensary can have markedly different amounts of both THC or CBD. An increasing ratio of CBD to THC tends to reduce the psychoactive side effects of THC. Therefore, the patient should be reminded with each new batch of cannabis he obtains to start with a low dose and titrate slowly upward to the desired effect. This should prevent the untoward psychoactive effects in the future.

A small percentage of patients elect to buy a device that can measure exactly the percentage of THC and CBD in the cannabis material.

There has been some suggestion of a potential for immuno-suppression from CBD because of its biphasic nature of CBD on immune-system cell lines. Lower doses of CBD are associated with stimulating response to the cell lines, but higher doses have an inhibitory effect.[12] Clinicians should be cautious when considering use of CBD in immunosuppressed patients.

In addition to mitigating the psychoactive side-effects of THC, CBD has been shown to mitigate THC-induced psychosis,[13–16]and THC-induced anxiety.[3,17]

The THC:CBD Ratio

The more recent research suggests that the clinician should think in terms of the THC, CBD, and the ratio of the two. The earlier studies focused on THC as the most relevant component of cannabis for medical purposes. The initial pharmaceutical agents in the mid-1980s were both synthetic forms of THC. However, the more recent studies are showing that CBD may well be the more significant pharmaceutical. It has significant effects, through the ECS and other biologic systems, on tumor suppression, inflammation, spasm, pain, and infertility. In addition, CBD mitigates the psychoactive euphoric effects of THC, making a combined THC/CBD medication more tolerable for clinical applications.[3] This observation of CBD's mitigating effects resulted in recreational marijuana users' genetically engineering cultivars of cannabis so they contained a lower percentage of CBD and a higher percentage of THC so that the euphoric effects were more pronounced.

At this juncture you should know that THC and CBD work on different symptoms and conditions, and that efficacy and adverse reactions vary when THC and CBD are in different ratios to each other. Often, increasing the percentage of CBD will protect against the psychoactive side-effects of THC.[3] The ratio of approximately 1:1 CBD to THC is the most studied, and it appears to be a good start for most conditions. Sativex is an oral spray that contains extracts of a patented cannabis cultivar; its CBD:THC ratio is approximately 1:1. This medication has been widely used around the world and is in stage III trials in the United States for FDA approval.

The primary care clinician needs to be very aware of the synergistic action between THC and CBD that produces analgesia, anti-inflammatory effects, and muscle relaxation. The majority of patients seek a physician's recommendation of medical cannabis for these beneficial effects. Others seek the anxiolytic effects and improved sense of well-being associated with cannabis use.

CBD, alone, on the other hand has a limited number of clinical effects but a much better side-effects profile, with none of the psychoactive effects of THC.

Medical Cannabis versus Recreational Cannabis

The concept of medical cannabis, as opposed to recreational cannabis, is for the most part a euphemism and not well defined. A practical definition would be that medical cannabis is any cannabis-based substance used to treat a medical condition. But most assuredly, this same cannabis-based substance can be used for recreational purposes if taken at the right dose and titration. Only the very low-THC cannabis does not have any recreational value.

A current law for medical cannabis being considered in Florida would make medical cannabis available, provided it is 5 percent or less THC. This is a typical political effort to diffuse the issue of medical versus recreational cannabis. Cannabis that had 5-percent potency was what was most available in prior decades and, if used for recreational purposes, has the desired euphoric effect. Thus, patients using cannabis for medical purposes might elect to use their cannabis for recreational purposes as well. So, in general, for clinicians, the concept of "purely" medical cannabis should be discarded. Currently, from a medical perspective there is very low-THC, high-CBD cannabis, which doesn't have any euphoric effects, and all other cannabis.

Pharmaceutical Cannabis Medicine

Although there are currently two pharmaceutical cannabinoid medications available—Marinol and Cesamet—these are not superior to currently available FDA-approved medications for the conditions for which they are recommended. It is unlikely that primary care clinicians will be prescribing Marinol or Cesamet. If and when Sativex is approved by the FDA, it will be the first prescription cannabis medication with effects similar to cannabis products currently available from cannabis dispensaries. It will likely be available at pharmacies and should be covered for several conditions by health insurance.

Patient Compliance to Medication

The medicinal effects of CBD have shown efficacy for a variety of conditions and symptoms, as discussed throughout this book. While there are effective pharmaceutical medications for most, if not all, of the conditions for which CBD can be used, probably the most obvious benefit is the excellent patient compliance to CBD treatment. Suboptimal adherence to many pharmaceuticals is often common and has adverse effects on clinical outcomes. CBD is widely tolerated and very safe. Forthcoming high-quality studies may support much wider use of medical cannabis as an opioid-sparing medication and for epilepsy, anxiety, psychosis, multiple sclerosis (MS), arthritis, and Parkinson's disease.

When to Recommend Medical Cannabis

Because of the wide variety of ways to ingest and titrate cannabinoids, the relatively low cost per dose, and the low risk of serious adverse effects or overdose, medical cannabis is used for a variety of medical conditions and symptoms that are on various states' lists of qualifying (approved) conditions. It must be kept in mind, however, that these lists are based on political or emotional reasons rather than hard science. Chapter 7 discusses the use of medical cannabis for each qualifying condition or symptom under state laws. It should be noted that the symptoms and conditions for which cannabis may be helpful are up to date and current as of the date of this publication. Several new and exciting basic science and clinical studies are soon to be released, and the results of the results reported will be added to the database of this burgeoning new area of medicine.

Typically, the primary care clinician will encounter three broad categories of clinical situations in which he or she will be required to make a decision about whether to recommend cannabis as the next step in treatment:

1. A patient comes to the clinician and asks to take medical cannabis for a common symptom such as chronic pain or anxiety.

2. The clinician recognizes a symptom or condition that may respond to cannabinoids.

3. All of the other generally recognized treatments for a condition or symptom have been tried without much or any success, and cannabis is a final option to add to the treatment regimen.

In all three scenarios, the clinician needs to determine if the condition or symptom is likely to be responsive to cannabinoids, if other more generally recognized treatments are likely to be superior to cannabinoids, if the psychoactive effects of the THC will impair or affect the patient adversely, and if there is a relative or absolute contraindication to use of cannabinoids.

As with opioids and benzodiazepines, the clinician needs to remain cognizant of the fact that some patients will feign symptoms or a condition in order to get cannabis to use for recreational purposes.

If cannabis is an appropriate next step in treatment, then the clinician writes a recommendation letter (*see* Appendix B for a prototype). The patient can take this to a medical marijuana dispensary to obtain medical cannabis. As for any medication, the clinician should have the patient return for regular follow-up visits to determine the medication's efficacy, compliance, and adverse effects.

Dosing Issues

How to dose cannabis is a fundamental issue among clinicians. Review of the literature over the decades reveals a wide range of doses and routes of administration. The literature is further obfuscated by the lack of good documentation of CBD:THC ratios and quality control of the percentage of the cannabinoids, as well as the fact that many of the studies were done with synthetic forms of THC from the pharmaceutical industry. Often, the studies cite "high-dose" or "low-dose" without a clear consensus about what these doses are. However, recent Dutch and Israeli epidemiologic studies have shown that patients who smoke cannabis use 600–1500 mg of plant material per day, divided over two to three doses, for symptom control.

Researchers have attempted to extrapolate weight-based doses from rodent studies to humans. However, this is not well founded due to the variance in bioavailability of the cannabinoids among mice and rats, as well as the difference in receptor prevalence in rodent organ systems.[18]

Studies of humans have shown great variation in bioavailability, depending on the route of administration. For CBD, the bioavailability may be as low as 6 percent if taken orally, due to the first-pass effect,[19] 34–46 percent if the intranasal route is used,[20] and 40 percent if administered through vaporization.[21] There may also be differences in CBD bioavailability through these routes, compared to that of THC.

Currently, unlike medications available as pharmaceuticals, almost all of the cannabis-based medications are not produced under the control of good manufacturing practices, which dictate strict labeling and purity requirements. This results in significant variation in doses of cannabinoids, even in the same product from the same manufacturer.[22]

At this point, dosing of cannabis plant-based medication, other than Sativex, cannot be considered scientifically based. The rule for titration—"start low, go slow"—should be applied. Remember, it can take 45–90 minutes for all of the effects (therapeutic and possible psychoactive effects) of the medication to become apparent, depending on the route of administration.

Adverse Effects

The side-effects from cannabis are strongly associated with the dose, how fast it is titrated and, most important, the route of administration: oral, inhalation by smoking, inhalation through vaporization, or dermal application. The thousands of by-products from smoked plant material lead to respiratory tract irritation and temporary cough. Vaporized and orally ingested cannabis do not have these side-effects. Prolonged use of smoked cannabis can result in increased cough and wheezing and chronic bronchitis. In addition, chronic obstructive pulmonary disease (COPD) has been reported as an adverse effect of cannabis smoking. The American Thoracic Society, in its publication *Smoking Marijuana and the Lungs* (www.thoracic.org /patients/patient-resources/resources/marijuana.pdf) stated that there is no clear association between cannabis smoking and lung or airway cancer. However, further research and evaluation of confounding factors, such as concomitant cigarette smoking, may require revision of this conclusion.

Other than acute anxiety or psychosis in a minority of patients, the main side-effects of THC and its metabolite 11-OH-THC are the psychoactive effects (e.g., mild euphoria, decreased short-term memory, cognitive deficits, impaired motor skills). In general, these tend to lessen over time and as the patient becomes more experienced in titrating the medicine. Short-term cognitive deficits from THC can be an unpleasant and dangerous side-effect, however. The cognitive impairment caused by THC can be as significant as alcohol-induced impairment, and motor vehicle accidents are reported to be 2.0–2.6 times more frequent after using cannabis.

THC may also have sympathomimetic effects, with associated vasodilation, causing conjunctival injection, mild orthostatic hypotension, and mild tachycardia.

Rapid absorption of higher doses of THC, usually through smoked or vaporized cannabis, can result in agitation or anxiety. This is especially true of patients who have never used cannabis, but this side-effect tends to quickly decrease with repeated use.

There is increasing evidence in the medical literature that THC can cause a psychotic break in up to 4 percent of patients, suggesting that the THC can trigger the manifestation of a tendency toward psychosis. This tendency should be addressed prior to recommending medical cannabis; if known or suggested by the patient's history, the clinician should closely monitor the patient during treatment.[23]

Cannabis use can cause transient cognitive impairment of short-term memory, concentration, attention, inhibition, and impulsivity. The research also supports heavy long-term use results in persistent cognitive effects.[24]

A cohort study of 1,000 persons followed from birth to age 38, found persistent neuropsychological deficits among adolescent cannabis users, years after cessation.[25] There is also evidence of permanent structural changes within the brain due to chronic use among adults.[26]

There is an interesting but rare condition associated with cannabis use: cannabis hyperemesis syndrome. This is recurrent, cyclic vomiting. Often the patient is not aware that the cannabis is the cause of the condition, and continues to increase the use of cannabis to try to treat the nausea and vomiting.[27] The clinician should advise the patient to immediately stop use of cannabis.

In addition, some patients report dose-related "highs" marked by easy laughing, elation, and heightened awareness. This is entirely due to ingestion of THC. Slower titration can reduce but not necessarily eliminate these "highs."

Routes of Delivery and Bioavailability

The bioavailability of cannabis varies greatly, depending on the route of administration. Smoked cannabis averages 30 percent bioavailability, with peak concentrations occurring 10 minutes after it is smoked. It is noted that the bioavailability following smoking ranges from 2 to 56 percent due, in part, to the wide variation of the smoking habits of individuals. In other words, variations in spacing of puffs, hold time, inhalation volume, and expectation of "drug reward" contribute to uncertainty about bioavailability.

With intranasal administration, the bioavailability is 34 to 46 percent; with vaporization, it is 40 percent; and with oral administration, it is only 4 to 12 percent due to the significant first-pass effect.[19] If orally administered via an edible or tincture, cannabis has an onset of action after 30–60 minutes and peak effect at 2–4 hours. With oral administration there is a large first-pass hepatic effect, and only 10 to 20 percent of the dose reaches the circulation. The psychoactive effects tend to last 4–6 hours.

Future pharmaceutical CBD, THC, and combinations of these will probably be in oromucosal and dermal preparations. Studies of Sativex suggest that it has 90 percent bioavailability, with rapid onset of action, when administered by the oromucosal route.[28] Cannabinoids are highly hydrophobic, making transdermal delivery challenging. There are no clinical studies of percutaneous absorption of cannabis-containing ointments, cream, or lotions. However, dermal patches have been shown to result in steady-state plasma concentrations within 1.4 hours, which was maintained for at least 48 hours. CBD was found to be 10 times more permeable than THC.

Overdose

Both THC and CBD are non-lethal regardless of the route of administration. This is because, unlike opioids and benzodiazepines, there are no endocannabinoid receptors in the brain stem, so there is no depressant effect on the respiratory system. However, as with opioids, benzodiazepines and several sedating medications, a sufficient dose of THC can cause extreme lethargy and cognitive impairment. This could result in a fatality from a driving accident or from being around dangerous equipment or in a dangerous environment.

Cannabis Dependence

The most recent studies of recreational cannabis users show that between 9 to 11 percent can become either physically or psychologically dependent on cannabis. Cannabis dependence is discussed in greater detail in Chapter 13.[29]

Precautions

THC may lower the seizure threshold. Seizures and seizure-like activity have been reported in patients who use cannabis.[30] If a patient has a history of seizure disorder, cannabis should be used with caution and close supervision. Medical cannabis should be discontinued if the patient develops seizures while taking the medication.

Because of the possibility of tachycardia, hypotension, hypertension or syncope, medical cannabis should be recommended with caution for patients with cardiac disorders.

Because of the possibility of a patient's developing psychological and physiologic dependence, psychiatric monitoring is recommended. However, physical addiction is uncommon. THC may aggravate pre-existing anxiety, depression, mania, or schizophrenia.[31]

Daily use of cannabis in patients with heptatitis C infection has been associated with increased steatosis and fibrosis. A study of 272 patients with chronic hepatitis C determined that daily cannabis use was a risk factor for progression of liver fibrosis.[32]

Cannabis has been linked in a dose-dependent manner with elevated rates of myocardial infarction and cardiac arrhythmias.[33]

Patients using concomitant CNS depressants, such as other medications or alcohol, can have additive or synergistic effects. These patients should be counseled about the risk this poses.

THC and CBD may interfere with other medications via metabolic and pharmacodynamic mechanisms. Both THC and CBD are highly protein-bound and may displace other protein-bound drugs. Patients concomitantly taking highly protein-bound medications should be monitored for changes in dosage requirements.

Summary: the Important Role of the Informed Clinician

Historically, most clinicians have had little or no training in the medicinal effects of cannabis and little background as to what to discuss about cannabis side-effects and dosing strategies. This is compounded by the dearth of high-quality medical literature on the subject. However, the growing number of conditions that can be treated with cannabis, and the growing body of basic science about the ECS and inter-patient variation in dose response, will make it imperative that clinicians take a more active role with their patients regarding the use of cannabis. Clinicians will have to schedule follow-up visits to discuss selection of the dose and how often to take it.

After absorbing the information in this book, the clinician can take a much more active role in determining the efficacy of cannabis therapy, not just writing a generic recommendation letter. If the clinician feels comfortable and adequately trained, cannabis that is higher in THC or CBD, or both, can be recommended. In addition, the clinician can recommend the starting dose, route of administration, dosing frequency, and ways to titrate to clinical effect, as well as effectively monitor patients. At follow-up visits, the clinician can determine if changes in the dose, route of delivery, and/or the cannabis formulation are necessary.

Notice that there is very little clinical information provided in this letter. Basically the clinician is certifying that the patient has one or more of the Qualifying Medical Conditions. The letter does not say which condition(s).

The patient, or his caregiver, can take that recommendation letter to a cannabis dispensary where the letter is used to permit medical cannabis to be dispensed. Or patients can use it in many states to grow their own limited number of cannabis plants. In many states the recommendation letter is used to put the patient in a medical cannabis registry.

Medical Marijuana Program WRITTEN DOCUMENTATION OF PATIENT'S MEDICAL RECORDS (Please Print)

Note to Attending Physician: This is not a mandatory form. If used, this form will serve as written documentation from the attending physician, stating that the patient has been diagnosed with a serious medical condition and that the medical use of marijuana is appropriate. A copy of this form must be filed in the attending physician's medical records for the patient. If the patient chooses to apply for a Medical Marijuana Identification card through the county health department or its designee, the agency will call your office to verify the information contained on this form.

Attending physician name California medical license number

Service mailing address (number, street) Office telephone number

( )

City State ZIP code Office fax number

( )

Licensed by (check one):

Medical Board of California Osteopathic Medical Board of California

                                                            is a patient under the medical care and supervision of the above Patient's name named physician who has diagnosed the patient with one or more of the following medical conditions:

1. Acquired Immune Deficiency Syndrome (AIDS) 2. Anorexia 3. Arthritis 4. Cachexia 5. Cancer 6. Chronic pain 7. Glaucoma 8. Migraine 9. Persistent muscle spasms, including, but not limited to, spasms associated with multiple sclerosis 10. Seizures, including, but not limited to, seizures associated with epilepsy 11. Severe nausea 12. Any other chronic or persistent medical symptom that either:

a. Substantially limits the ability of the person to conduct one or more major life activities as defined in the Americans with

    Disabilities Act of 1990. b. If not alleviated, may cause serious harm to the patient's safety or physical or mental health

ATTENDING PHYSICIAN STATEMENT:

This patient has been diagnosed with one or more of the foregoing medical conditions and the use of medical marijuana is appropriate.

Name of physician or physician staff completing this form Telephone number Date

Original—Patient Copy—Patient's File

Figure 9-1 Example of Recommendation Letter

Patient Who Has Never Before Used Cannabis

A patient is about to be started on cannabis therapy with a cultivar of cannabis that is high in THC. He is naïve to the use of cannabis. What side-effect should you spend extra time discussing with the patient, since he is naïve to its use? What should you explain to him, that a patient not naïve to cannabis might already understand?

Discussion: Naïve patients who use any form of cannabis, or THC medication, need to be advised of the often potent psychoactive effects of euphoria, uncontrolled laughter, and spatial disorientation. The first few times someone experiences these side-effects can be quite alarming. The patient should be strongly cautioned about the psychoactive effects and how to minimize them by starting with very low doses and titrating the dose slowly to get the medical effect, with minimal side-effects.

The naïve patient can be advised that, with practice and experience, the psychoactive effects will lessen, and a true biologic tolerance to the psychoactive effects usually develops in a couple of weeks.

A patient with prior experience using cannabis will usually understand the concept of titrating the dosing of the medication, to gradually obtain symptom control. The clinician will usually have to explain titrating the dosing in some detail to the naïve patient, and will have to advise them to allow a week or two, until they are experienced in titrating to minimize side-effects, and maximize symptom control.

Patients Without Health Insurance Coverage

Another aspect of treating a patient with medical cannabis is the fact that the cannabis, supplies, and probably the pharmacogenetic testing are not paid for by health insurance. Although the clinician visit and testing associated with the diagnosis will be covered by health insurance, the medication and supplies are not. This is because of legal issues surrounding medical cannabis, and the fact that the medication is not FDA approved. If the DEA and FDA change cannabis to a different scheduled drug, then insurance-related reimbursement issues may resolve. Because of DEA and other federal banking laws, it is likely that the patient will have to pay for the cannabis and supplies with cash. Credit cards and checks are usually not taken. Again, simple changes in the banking rules can alleviate this situation quickly.

Pediatric, Geriatric, and Pregnant Patients

THC has not been studied in pediatric populations. Caution should be observed when using THC in pediatric populations because of issues with the psychoactive effects. In addition, long-term neurocognitive effects are suspected. CBD is used regularly in pediatric populations with no reported issues. Geriatric patients may be more sensitive to the sympathomimetic and psychoactive effects of THC. In addition, increased somnolence and dizziness may increase risk of falls in this population. It is prudent to start at the lowest starting doses and titrate up very slowly.

THC has not been well studied in pregnant women. It is Category C for pregnancy risks based on studies in rodents. It should be used only if the potential benefits justify the potential risks.

THC and CBD have not been studied in nursing mothers. Cannabinoids are fat soluble and can transfer in low doses through breast milk.

Patients with Cancer or At Risk for Cancer Carcinogenesis

There are at least 33 constituents present in both cannabis smoke and tobacco smoke that are listed as carcinogens.

Cannabis smoke is at best weakly mutagenic, and as such may promote cancer development. An excellent summary of the available evidence on the carcinogenesis of cannabis was published by the California Environmental Protection Agency in 2009 [http://oehha.ca.gov/prop65/hazard_ident/pdf_zip /FinalMJsmokeHID.pdf]. They found 27 high-quality studies and several case reports on the topic of cannabis and carcinogensis. Cigarette smoking was a major confounder in most of the studies. There were several studies that report statistically significant associations between cannabis smoking and cancer of the head and neck, lung, bladder, brain, and testis. There were also epidemiologic studies supporting a link between parental cannabis smoking and childhood cancer, especially leukemia. However, the evidence is limited and inconclusive as to whether smoking cannabis increases the risk of any cancer.

Patients Who Are Trying to Conceive

Long-term use of cannabis may have an adverse impact of reproduction. It has been shown to disrupt menstrual cycles, suppress oogenesis, and impair embryo implantation and fetal development.[34] It also affects testosterone levels and spermatogenesis.

CHAPTER 10

Pharmacogenetic Testing

I n the past, because the staff at marijuana dispensaries have regular visits with their patients and deal intimately with the efficacy and side-effects from the cannabis, the clinician had often not felt involved with patient management after the requisite recommendation letter has been written. This should not be the case.

The burgeoning use of pharmacogenetic testing prior to starting long-term medications in naïve patients is changing the physician-patient relationship for the better. There is a small but growing number of medications for which pharmacogenetic testing is required before they are prescribed. The number of medications for which pharmacogenetic testing is "recommended" has become much larger and is growing.

What is Pharmacogenetics?

Pharmacogenetics is the study of individual variation in the genetic sequence related to drug response. Pharmocogenetic testing identifies various alternative and mutant forms of alleles of genes for enzymes involved in the metabolism of medications.

A gene is a section of DNA that determines a certain trait. When there is more than one form of the gene, these various mutations of the gene are called *alleles*. An allele is one of two or more forms of a gene, which arise by mutation. Since chromosomes occur in pairs, there are two alleles for each gene. Since each chromosome comes from a different parent, there can be two of the same allele (homozygous) and two different alleles (heterozygous). There are often dozens of different alleles for any particular gene. When it comes to medications, the different alleles cause decreased metabolism, increased or "super" increased metabolism, or entirely inactive metabolism. The consequences of these variations in allele metabolism can cause the drug to act very differently in some patients, compared to most of the population, who have "average" metabolic effects. Sometimes, the consequences of the different metabolic responses to allele variations are not as simple as needing to lower or raise the dose of the medication. Certain mutant alleles in the fatty acid amide hydrolase (FAAH) system can lead to greatly increased risk for addictive behavior with certain prescribed medications, such as THC.

Predicting Response to Drugs

These different alleles can be used to help determine if a patient is more likely to have a good response or an adverse effect from the use of the medication being tested. Therefore, appropriate and carefully interpreted pharmacogenetic testing of individuals can help personalize their drug choices, and assist the clinician with starting doses of cannabinoids in first-time users of medical cannabis.

Only a small number of tests for specific gene alleles have been shown to be helpful for cannabinoids. Some of the more forward-thinking clinical laboratories around the country are bundling these tests to assist doctors who are prescribing cannabis. As with any newly developing technology, the doctor should select high-quality, reputable, and certified laboratories to test their specimens.

Some of these same alleles are also involved with the metabolism of a wide variety of other medications. The list keeps growing at a rapidly expanding rate.

Cytochrome P450 system

The cytochrome P450 system, abbreviated CYP, is the most important system involved with cannabis metabolism in the body. It accounts for 75 percent of the enzymes involved with medication metabolism. There are 60 CYP genes; however, only a few are tested for when prescribing cannabis. Each gene is named CYP plus a number- and letter-combination to show to which subgroup it is assigned (e.g., CYP1B1).

The CYP genes are involved with catalyzing a vast number of reactions, mostly in the liver, and primarily in steroid synthesis and detoxification. Some detoxify medicinal compounds to facilitate excretion, while others turn inactive compounds into active pharmacologic agents.

If a CYP enzyme metabolizes a drug slowly, the drug stays longer in the body. If it metabolizes a drug more quickly, a higher dose may be needed to have an effect.

There is increased biosynthesis of CYP enzymes in response to increased demand, in a feedback loop. Many medications and other substances, such as alcohol, can lead to increased biosynthesis of a particular CYP enzyme, making it more metabolically active.

This type of testing has become readily available, although at this time the costs and insurance reimbursement are still barriers to use. An expanding group of reputable laboratories can process a simple buccal sample in a few days. Because of the nature of genetic finger-printing in quality laboratories, these tests usually have 99-percent sensitivity and 99-percent specificity.

CYP2D6

There are several CYP enzymes that can be tested for prior to use of cannabinoids. The first one to be discussed is CYP2D6. This enzyme acts on 25 percent of all known drugs, including cannabinoids. Drugs such as opioids, selective serotonin reuptake inhibitors (SSRIs), sildenafil, tricyclic antidepressants, and beta-blockers are some of the drugs metabolized by this enzyme. It is important to note that CBD is a powerful inhibitor of CYP2D6, and two other CYP enzymes. Therefore, it potentiates the effects of drugs that are metabolized by CYP2D6. This should be carefully considered when choosing high-CBD strains of cannabis.

About 7–14 percent of the general population have the "slow" version of the CYP2D6 enzyme, 7 percent have the "superfast", and 35 percent of the population are "carriers", wherein one of the two alleles is nonfunctional. Patients with the slow version of CYP2D6 require a lower starting dose and less frequent

AIBioTech®
AMERICAN INTERNATIONAL BIOTECHNOLOGY, LLC

Drug Metabolism Test Requisition
All blue and yellow highlighted fields are required. Failure to complete these fields will delay patient results. For questions contact Account Support at:
1.888.785.8789 | accountsupport@aibiotech.com

Collection Date (MM/DD/YYYY):	Collection Time (AM/PM):	Sample Collected By:	Requisition Completed By:

Physician Information

Physician Name:		Practice Name:	Office Phone:	
Practice Address:		City:	State:	Zip:

Physician/Authorizing Medical Professional's Signature: By signing this test requisition, I certify that I have obtained informed consent (as outlined on the reverse of this form) from the patient as required by any applicable state or federal laws with respect to each test ordered. If patient signature is not located on the requisition, it is indicated to AIBioTech® that the physician has obtained written informed consent which is documented in the patient records. I attest that the diagnosis codes selected below are accurate and supported by information in the patient records. I also understand that each genetic panel may include a combination of the following tests: CYP2D6, CYP2C19, CYP2C9, VKORC1, CYP3A4/3A5, ApoE, Factor II, Factor V and MTHFR (see test listing on reverse of this form). NOTE: Physician should make and keep a copy of this requisition for the patient records.

Physician/Medical Professional's Signature (Original signatures only, stamped or photocopied signatures cannot be accepted and will delay patient results.):

X_____

Patient Information

☐ See attached patient demographic sheet. (If a patient demographic sheet is attached, patient name and date of birth fields must still be completed.)

Patient Name:		Patient Date of Birth (MM/DD/YYYY):	Patient Gender: ☐ Male ☐ Female	
Patient Address:		City:	State:	Zip:	Phone:

Patient Race/Ethnic Identification:
☐ African-American ☐ Asian ☐ Caucasian ☐ Hispanic ☐ Other _____

Patient Consent Signature: I authorize the release of medical information related to this service for submission of personalized reports to my healthcare providers and insurance carriers. I request that payment of authorized benefits be made on my behalf to AIBioTech®. If my current policy prohibits direct payment to AIBioTech®, I agree to receive the funds and relinquish them to AIBioTech® as payment towards charges for services rendered. I also acknowledge that I will be liable for payment of deductible, co-payment and/or co-insurance as assigned by my healthcare insurer and may be responsible for charges for laboratory services that are not covered by my healthcare insurer. I authorize AIBioTech® to appeal insurance claims on my behalf. My signature below constitutes my acknowledgement that the benefits, risks, and limitations of this testing have been explained to my satisfaction by a qualified health professional and as described on the reverse of this form.

Patient Signature (Required by insurance):   Patient Social Security Number:

X_____

Test Request	**Diagnosis (ICD-9) Codes**					**Insurance and Payment**

Check the box beside the desired panel, based on patient's medical needs:
☐ PersonaGene™ Panel (includes all panels below)
OR
Select up to three of the panels below.
☐ CardioloGene™ Panel
☐ Pain Management Panel
☐ PsychiaGene™ Panel
☐ UroloGene™ Panel
(See test listing on reverse of this form)

Use the appropriate ICD-9 codes to indicate medical diagnosis. Write in codes not listed on the blank lines below. Insurance companies require codes to the highest level possible using fourth and fifth digits. For a short list of ICD-9 codes and descriptions, refer to the back of this form.

☐ 272.0	☐ 296.51	☐ 401.9	☐ 411.1	☐ 724.4
☐ 296.30	☐ 296.52	☐ 410.00	☐ 411.89	☐ 726.10
☐ 296.31	☐ 296.60	☐ 410.10	☐ 413.0	☐ 729.5
☐ 296.32	☐ 296.61	☐ 410.20	☐ 427.31	☐ 995.20
☐ 296.50	☐ 296.62	☐ 411.0	☐ 724.2	☐ V58.69

Photocopy of both sides of patient insurance card(s) must be included.
Patient signature and social security number are required by some insurance companies. If an ABN is required please attach it to this form
☐ Medicare ☐ Self Pay
☐ Insurance

Sample Collection Method
Buccal swab (swab rubbed firmly in each cheek and under gum)

Patient List of Medications

Check the boxes for the patient's medications here for a PersonaGene™ Medication Report. A current medications list may also be attached from the patient's record. Results will only be available for the medications listed below.

☐ Decline PersonaGene™ Medication Report

☐ Clopidogrel (Plavix)	☐ Methadone (Dolophine)	☐ Flurbiprofen (Ansaid)	☐ Carisoprodol (Soma)	☐ Venlafaxine (Effexor, Effexor XR)
☐ Warfarin (Coumadin)	☐ Codeine	☐ Ibuprofen (Advil, Motrin)	☐ Meperidine (Demerol)	☐ Aripiprazole (Abilify, Abilify Discmelt)
☐ Carvedilol (Coreg)	☐ Dihydrocodeine (Synalgos)	☐ Indomethacin (Indocin)	☐ Citalopram (Celexa)	☐ Haloperidol (Haldol)
☐ Metoprolol (Lopressor)	☐ Morphine	☐ Lornoxicam (Xefo)	☐ Escitalopram (Lexapro)	☐ Pimozide (Orap)
☐ Propranolol	☐ Hydrocodone	☐ Meloxicam (Mobic)	☐ Sertraline (Zoloft)	☐ Diazepam (Valium)
☐ Timolol	☐ Oxycodone	☐ Naproxen (Aleve, Anaprox, Naprosyn)	☐ Amitriptyline (Elavil)	☐ Clonazepam (Klonopin)
☐ Ticagrelor (Brilinta)	☐ Tramadol (Ultracet)	☐ Nortriptyline (Pamelor)	☐ Atomoxetine (Strattera)
☐ Atorvastatin (Lipitor)	☐ Fentanyl Acediofenac	☐ Piroxicam (Feldene)	☐ Clomipramine (Anafranil)	☐ Tetrabenazine (Xenazine)
☐ Lovastatin (Mevacor)	☐ Celecoxib (Celebrex)	☐ Suprofen (Profenal)	☐ Fluoxetine (Prozac)
☐ Simvastatin (Zocor)	☐ Diclofenac (Cataflam, Voltaren)	☐ Tenoxicam (Mobiflex)	☐ Duloxetine (Cymbalta)

AIB-RQ022-0814F

Figure 10-1 Example of a Pharmacogenetic Requisition Form (page 1)

titration because the ingested medicine will tend to accumulate in the blood faster than an average patient.

Patients with the superfast version of the CYP2D6 enzyme tend not to respond to usual doses of cannabinoids because the enzyme metabolizes the medication very quickly. This will be especially obvious with orally ingested edibles and tinctures, because of their first-pass effect from the liver.

Code	Diagnosis Description	Code	Diagnosis Description	Code	Diagnosis Description
272.0	Hypercholesterolemia, pure	296.62	Bipolar I Disorder, Most Recent Episode (or Current) Mixed, Moderate	410.70	Subendocardial Infarction Episode of Care Unspecified
296.30	Major Depressive Affective Disorder Recurrent Episode Unspecified Degree	296.63	Bipolar I Disorder, Most Recent Episode (or Current) Mixed, Severe, Without Mention of Psychotic Behavior	410.80	Acute Myocardial Infarction of Other Specified Sites Episode of Care Unspecified
296.31	Major Depressive Affective Disorder Recurrent Episode Mild Degree	296.64	Bipolar I Disorder, Most Recent Episode (or Current) Mixed, Severe, Specified As With Psychotic Behavior	410.90	Acute Myocardial Infarction of Unspecified Site Episode of Care Unspecified
296.32	Major Depressive Affective Disorder Recurrent Episode Moderate Degree	296.65	Bipolar I Disorder, Most Recent Episode (or Current) Mixed, In Partial Or Unspecified Remission	411.0	Postmyocardial Infarction Syndrome
296.33	Major Depressive Affective Disorder Recurrent Episode Severe Degree without Psychotic Behavior	296.66	Bipolar I Disorder, Most Recent Episode (or Current) Mixed, In Full Remission	411.1	Intermediate Coronary Syndrome
296.34	Major Depressive Affective Disorder Recurrent Episode Severe Degree Specified as with Psychotic Behavior	296.65	Bipolar I Disorder, Most Recent Episode (or Current) Mixed, In Partial Or Unspecified Remission	411.81	Acute Coronary Occlusion without Myocardial Infarction
296.35	Major Depressive Affective Disorder Recurrent Episode In Partial or Unspecified Remission	296.66	Bipolar I Disorder, Most Recent Episode (or Current) Mixed, In Full Remission	411.89	Other Acute and Subacute Forms of Ischemic Heart Disease Other
296.36	Major Depressive Affective Disorder Recurrent Episode In Full Remission	311	Depressive Disorder Not Elsewhere Classified	413.0	Angina Decubitus
296.50	Bipolar I Disorder, Most Recent Episode (or Current) Depressed, Unspecified	333.4	Huntington's Chorea	413.1	Prinzmetal Angina
296.51	Bipolar I Disorder, Most Recent Episode (or Current) Depressed, Mild	401.9	Hypertension, unspecified	413.9	Other and Unspecified Angina Pectoris
296.52	Bipolar I Disorder, Most Recent Episode (or Current) Depressed, Moderate	410.00	Acute Myocardial Infarction of Anterolateral Wall Episode of Care Unspecified	427.31	Atrial fibrillation
296.53	Bipolar I Disorder, Most Recent Episode (or Current) Depressed, Severe, Without Mention Of Psychotic Behavior	410.10	Acute Myocardial Infarction of Other Anterior Wall Episode of Care Unspecified	724.20	Lumbago
296.54	Bipolar I Disorder, Most Recent Episode (or Current) Depressed, Severe, Specified As With Psychotic Behavior	410.20	Acute Myocardial Infarction of Inferolateral Wall Episode of Care Unspecified	724.40	Thoracic or Lumbosacral neuritis or radiculitis, unspecified
296.55	Bipolar I Disorder, Most Recent Episode (or Current) Depressed, In Partial Or Unspecified Remission	410.30	Acute Myocardial Infarction of Inferoposterior Wall Episode of Care Unspecified	729.5	Pain in limb
296.56	Bipolar I Disorder, Most Recent Episode (or Current) Depressed, In Full Remission	410.40	Acute Myocardial Infarction of Other Inferior Wall Episode of Care Unspecified	788.41	Urinary frequency
296.60	Bipolar I Disorder, Most Recent Episode (or Current) Mixed, Unspecified	410.50	Acute Myocardial Infarction of Other Lateral Wall Episode of Care Unspecified	995.20	Unspecified adverse effect of unspecified drug, medicinal and biological substance
296.61	Bipolar I Disorder, Most Recent Episode (or Current) Mixed, Mild	410.60	True Posterior Wall Infarction Episode of Care Unspecified	V58.69	High-risk medication, long-term use

Sample Submission Instructions

1. Complete required information on this requisition form (highlighted areas and test required.) Make a copy of this form and keep it in the patient's record.

2. Legibly write patient's last name and DOB on the back of the AIBioTech® coin envelope.

3. Place envelope containing buccal swabs (swabs rubbed firmly in each cheek), test requisition and insurance information into large AIBioTech® envelope and seal.

4. Affix large preprinted return label to supplied return shipping package, keeping small label for your records.

5. Place large AIBioTech® envelope into the supplied return shipping package and send to AIBioTech®.

Informed Consent Information

Submission of an order for any genetic test listed on this requisition constitutes acknowledgement by the ordering physician and patient that:

1. Each genetic test may include a combination of the following tests: CYP2D6, CYP2C19, CYP2C9, VKORC1, CYP3A4/3A5, ApoE, Factor II, Factor V and MTHFR.

2. The ordering physician has obtained written informed consent as required by any applicable state or federal laws with respect to each test ordered. We provide an informed consent form at http://www.aibiotech.com/physicians/account-support-forms for your convenience. A copy of the written informed consent is not required by the laboratory to process the sample.

3. Patient authorization has been obtained permitting AIBioTech® to report the results of each test ordered directly to the physician.

4. DNA results may:

   a. Diagnose whether or not a patient has a condition or is at risk for developing a condition

   b. Indicate whether or not a patient is a carrier for a condition

   c. Predict another family member has or is at risk for developing a condition

   d. Predict another family member is a carrier of a condition

   e. Be indeterminate due to technical limitations or familial genetic patterns.

5. This DNA test is specific only for drug metabolism and cardiovascular risk factors and will not detect all causative mutations.

6. The significance of a positive and a negative test result based on a patient's family history has been explained.

7. Although DNA testing usually yields precise information, several sources of error are possible. These include, but are not limited to, clinical misdiagnosis of the condition, sample misidentification, and inaccurate information regarding family relationships.

8. Test results are released to the ordering health care provider or those entitled to them by state and local laws.

9. AIBioTech® is authorized under Clinical Laboratory Improvement Amendments (CLIA) to perform high-complexity testing. The results are not intended to be used as the sole means for clinical diagnosis or patient management decisions.

10. Genetic counseling is recommended prior to, as well as following, genetic testing.

11. The requested DNA test may contain additional quality control (QC) markers that are reviewed and the data retained from specific genetic locations. These QC markers may be used for specific quality control steps of the testing process. In addition, de-identified, extracted DNA may be used as blinded validation or specimen for research and development. No additional results beyond the genetic tests requested and the QC markers will be interpreted on this sample. Following testing and QC, the sample will be destroyed.

12. The patient acknowledges that they may obtain a copy of their written informed consent form from the physician and that test information sheets are available at www.aibiotech.com/patients.

	CYP2D6	CYP2C19	CYP2C9	VKORC1	CYP3A4	CYP3A5	ApoE	Factor II	Factor V	MTHFR
PersonaGene™ Panel	×	×	×	×	×	×	×	×	×	×
CardioloGene™ Panel	×	×	×	×	×	×	×	×	×	×
Pain Management Panel	×	×	×		×	×				
PsychiaGene™ Panel	×	×	×		×					
UroloGene™ Panel	×	×	×		×					

AIB-RQ022-0814F

Figure 10-1 Example of a Pharmacogenetic Requisition Form (page 2)

CYP3A4

The next most useful enzyme to test for is CYP3A4. This enzyme is the most prevalent CYP enzyme in the liver. It acts on 50 percent of all known drugs, including cannabinoids. While CYP3A4 inactivates many drugs, some are actually activated by this enzyme. A wide variety of medications, as well as grapefruit juice and CBD, are strong inhibitors of this enzyme, which may amplify or weaken the response to the drugs that it impacts. It is beyond the scope of this book to list the drugs that CYP3A4 acts on, but the list would include many of the most common drugs used in clinical practice.

H1CYP2C19

CYP2C19 acts on between 5–10 percent of all known drugs, including cannabinoids. Drugs such as SSRIs, tricyclic antidepressants, barbituates, and proton-pump inhibitors (PPIs) are metabolized by CYP2C19.

H1CYP2CP

CYP2CP acts on 15 percent of all known drugs, including cannabinoids. It is important because many of the drugs that it metabolizes have a narrow therapeutic window. These drugs include nonsteroidal anti-inflammatory drugs (NSAIDs), phenytoin, angiotensin, glipizide, and warfarin. The "slow" version of this enzyme can result in unexpected elevated blood levels in response to normal doses of cannabis and to drug-drug interactions with potentially lethal co-administered effects.

CYP1A2

CYP1A2 acts on 5–10 percent of all known drugs, including cannabinoids. It is induced by a wide variety of vegetables and certain spices, including curry. Some of the more common medications that it metabolizes are caffeine, theophylline, ciprofloxacin, and clozepine.

Other enzymes, besides the CYP enzymes, are involved with cannabinoid metabolism. However, pharmacogenetic testing for these is not recommended at this time.

Separate from knowledge of which alleles are present in an individual patient's genetic code, the clinician needs to take a thorough history to determine if other medications or the use of alcohol are stimulating increased activity of the metabolic systems, which likewise would have a significant effect on how cannabis is metabolized and would affect the patient's dose or frequency of dosing. This also holds true with regard to frequent cannabis users and changes in the metabolism of other medications. For example, regular cannabis use may accelerate the metabolism of theophylline or slow the metabolism of beta-blockers. Synergistic effects may accrue from the concomitant use of cannabis and opioids.

Screening for Potential Cannabis Dependence

Cannabis use has long been considered to be addictive, which has contributed to its bad reputation as a dangerous drug. Indeed, the available evidence suggests that about 9–11 percent of people who try cannabis for recreational purposes may become dependent on it.[29] There is some evidence that a very small percentage of users may become physically addicted to THC.

This dependence is associated with a well-described syndrome characterized by a pattern of compulsive use of cannabis and sometimes physiologic dependence on it, with increasing dosage tolerance or symptoms of withdrawal. Other more specific symptoms include impaired motivation and memory, anxiety, reality distortion, and social withdrawal.

The DSM-5 Diagnostic Codes Related to Substance Use Disorders (May 2013) has the following two diagnostic codes: 304.30 for cannabis dependence and 305.20 for cannabis abuse.

New research has uncovered two different phenotypes of enzymes that are markers for an increased risk of dependence. Testing for these phenotypes in a naïve patient prior to using medical cannabis may become standard clinical practice in the future. Specifically, it would be helpful for genetic markers in individuals who are more likely to develop a craving for cannabis, have withdrawal symptoms, or have increased sensitivity to cannabinoids' euphoric effects.

(http://pubs.niaaa.nih.gov/publications/arh312/111-118.pdf).

C385A

Fatty acid amide hydrolase (FAAH) is an enzyme that inactivates anandamide, an endogenous agonist of CB1 receptors. Studies have shown that CB1 binding modulates mescocorticolimbic dopamine release, which is very important in several facets of addiction. The C385A variant of FAAH has been shown to be associated with withdrawal after abstinence.[35] Further study of this variant is necessary before C385A testing can be recommended.

(The ECS and cannabinoid receptors are discussed in detail in Chapter 3.) Another promising area for genetic testing is for cannabinoid receptor 1 (CB1) variants. At this time, the studies are suggestive but inconclusive about an association between certain CB1 variants and an increased risk of cannabis dependence and cannabis-related uncovering of schizophrenia. However, recent human studies[36,37] of the AKT1 gene, which is involved with dopamine signaling, have shown that carrying one variant of this gene greatly increases the chance of developing a psychotic disorder if cannabis is used. The risk doubled with infrequent cannabis use, and it increased seven-fold in daily users of cannabis.

Catechol-O-methyltransferase (COMT) is involved in the metabolism of dopamine, epinephrine, and norepinephrine. It is especially important for dopamine regulation in the prefrontal cortex. Several drugs, including THC, target COMT to alter its activity and therefore the availability of catecholamines. Early scientific evidence suggests that COMT gene polymorphism may play a role in the pathogenesis of schizophrenia related to the use of cannabis.[38] Again, the evidence is still not convincing enough to support testing for COMT variants prior to initiation of medical cannabis.

Pharmacogenetics is a rapidly evolving field of basic science and clinical science research. In the future, new discoveries and changes in the understanding of genetic variants and drug metabolism may make genetic testing a necessity of clinical practice.

Insurance coding and reimbursement issues related to pharmacogenetics testing are discussed in the chapter on insurance issues.

Chronic Pain in Patient Who Has Never Used Cannabis

A patient presents to you whom is naïve to cannabis. She is on a variety of other medications for her chronic pain, including an SSRI and frequent daily doses of opioids. She is to be started medical cannabis that is high in CBD and low in THC. With your recommendation, what pharmacogenetic issues should you be concerned about? What will the adverse effects be if pharmacogenetic testing shows that she has the slow version of the CYP2D6 enzyme?

Discussion: This is a case in which the patient is on a number of medicines that are processed by the CYP2D6 enzyme. CBD is known to depress the activity of CYP2D6 and to potentiate the effects of drugs metabolized by CYP2D6, which include opioids and SSRIs.

In this scenario, chronic CBD use by the patient could depress the CYP2D6 enzyme and result in higher concentrations of opioids and SSRIs in the blood than their concentrations before cannabis therapy is initiated. This is especially true for the opioids because of their narrow therapeutic window. Pharmacogenetic testing is important for this patient.

CHAPTER 11

Writing Recommendation Letters for Cannabis Use

In regard to recommending cannabis for treatment, Fitzcharles and colleagues in 2014 wrote, "Simply acceding to patient demands for a treatment on the basis of popular advocacy, without comprehensive knowledge of any agent, does not adhere to the ethical standards of medical practice . . . any recommended therapy requires proof of concept by sound scientific study that attests to both efficacy and safety."[153]

A 2013 summary of the evidence[2] states that all but the most biased reviews on the topic of using cannabis for medical conditions, conclude with statements such as, "Medical cannabis appears to have some benefit in patients with certain conditions."

Most clinicians have never had formal training in the clinical use of cannabis. Even after medical cannabis is clearly legalized and medical board policies and legal issues are clarified to help practicing clinicians, a number of clinicians may hesitate to recommend cannabis. As mentioned in the Introduction, even in Colorado, where medical cannabis has been legal for over a decade, only about 10 percent of physicians are recommending cannabis to their patients.

One of the barriers to a higher proportion of clinicians recommending cannabis is the need for specific education on how to recommend cannabis for appropriate conditions and symptoms and, of course, how to manage and conduct follow-up evaluation of patients who are using medical cannabis.

At this time, it is illegal under FDA and DEA regulations for a clinician to actually prescribe cannabis. This is true even in states where medical cannabis has been legalized. Since cannabis is a Schedule I drug, according to federal regulations, medical use of the drug is prohibited. So, the clinician must write a recommendation letter that can be taken to the cannabis dispensary. The recommendation letter requirements vary from state to state. Appendix B contains an example of the official state of California letter. The format of the letter will be slightly different in each state. The clinician is advised to check the current state regulations on recommendation letters.

Basic Procedure

Remember, recommendation letters are analogous to prescriptions and should be written after each follow-up visit.

Often, the patient will come to the clinician to specifically ask for a recommendation letter for a particular condition. Prior to deciding to recommend cannabis for the treatment of the condition, the clinician should take a sufficient history to determine that other more generally recognized treatments have been tried but have not been adequately effective. If the clinician finds that not all of the other available treatments have been tried, he or she should explain why these should be tried first. The patient can be told that, while cannabis may be appropriate for the condition, it is beneficial to try other remedies with fewer side-effects and more controlled delivery vehicles, such as tablets and capsules, prior to recommending cannabis. The paucity of research on cannabis for the condition can also be mentioned.

The personal expense of using cannabis medication should be brought up, as this may be a real barrier. The patient should be made aware that although the clinic visits and associated lab work are covered by health insurance, the cannabis medicine, supplies, and paraphernalia are not and that the paraphernalia can easily cost $50 to $200 to start, and the medicine $100 to $200 a month.

If it is determined that medical cannabis is the appropriate next step, then the clinician writes a formal recommendation letter. This letter can be taken to a dispensary where, in most states, it provides the patient with a Medical Marijuana Card, which looks something like a driver's license. This card will allow the patient to carry specific amounts of cannabis products or to grow a specific number of cannabis plants. Also, in some states, the patient will then be put into a registry database which can easily be searched by professionals with a need to know.

It is important to note that the template of the California recommendation letter in the appendix of this book is provided as a guideline on what information needs to be in the recommendation letter; it is usually not a mandatory template format.

The important aspect of the letter is that it contains the patient-identification information, the clinician who is the point of contact, and the licensing information. The letter should have either an expiration date for the recommendation and/or a patient re-evaluation date.

The conditions or symptoms for which medical cannabis is legal under state laws keeps expanding. Each state usually documents these on its template letter. It is generally not necessary to document the particular condition for which cannabis is being recommended.

So far, a couple dozen states have some form of legalized medical cannabis, and the number is increasing annually. The clinician is advised to check with his or her state medical board for current rules and policies on recommendation letters, recognized diagnoses and conditions, and appropriate frequency of follow-up visits.

The recommendation letter has very little to do with the clinical management of the patient. The letter certifies more or less a diagnosis for which medical cannabis is qualified for use in that state. If possible, it is best for the clinician to certify the patient at the initial visit for only two to four weeks so that the patient will be required to return for follow-up evaluation of the efficacy, adverse effects, and possible development of cannabis dependence syndrome.

At each follow-up visit, the clinician should produce a new recommendation letter that allows the patient to purchase medical cannabis from dispensaries until the date of the next follow-up visit.

Follow-up visits and clinical monitoring of cannabis patients are discussed in detail in Chapter 12.

When the patient takes the letter to a cannabis dispensary, the dispensary staff will educate the patient about the options for using medical cannabis, provide advice on routes of administration, and will sell the individual the cannabis medication and paraphernalia.

Some patients will not want to use a dispensary, but rather wish to grow their own cannabis plants. In this situation, a recommendation letter that lasts only two to four weeks would not be very helpful, since it takes cannabis plants three to four months to grow from seed to budding plant. In this scenario, the clinician should write a recommendation letter for a six-month period, as this will give the patient time to purchase the appropriate seeds from the dispensary, grow them until they bud, and allow time for the patient to process the cannabis buds and determine if use of the cannabis has beneficial medicinal benefits.

Taking a More Active Role

Clinicians with adequate training and experience in treating patients with medical cannabis may start taking a more active role in managing the type of cannabis product, dosing, and route of administration. The clinician who takes a more active role gives the patient a document separate from the recommendation letter, with suggestions to the dispensary staff about type of cannabis product, dosing, and route of drug delivery. However, these facts are not included in the recommendation letter. This letter is only for the administrative and registry purposes of the state.

Hopefully, after a clinician reads this book or takes a training course on medical cannabis, he or she will be inclined to take a much more active role in the use of medical cannabis for the condition, including visiting local dispensaries to learn about what they have available and to create an open dialogue with the dispensary staff.

Unlike highly regulated, closely supervised pharmacies, dispensaries can vary in many ways. In addition, the amount of documentation is quite limited, compared to clinicians' medical records. The education, certification, and supervision of the dispensary staff is variable and limited. Only a trained and qualified clinician will have the necessary training, experience, and diagnostic expertise to professionally manage the use of medical cannabis.

Format for Recommendation Letters

*You are in a rush and want to quickly write a recommenda-
tion letter to start cannabis for a patient. You consider using a
nearby prescription pad to write the recommendation. What
would be wrong with this?*

Discussion: Under federal law, writing a formal prescription
for plant-based cannabis is illegal in every state. At this time,
cannabis is still a Schedule I Controlled Substance, and the
FDA's position is that there are no legitimate medical uses for
cannabis. However, because cannabinoid pharmaceuticals
such as Marinol and Cesamet are Schedule II and III substances, they can be prescribed.

Using a prescription sheet to write a recommendation
letter could be construed as prescribing cannabis and should
not be done.

CHAPTER 12

Monitoring Cannabis Medication

O ver the past 18 years during which medical cannabis has been legal in various states, the clinician has often relegated patient monitoring to the dispensaries and registered caregivers. The medication management has been informally delegated to the dispensary staff. This has been for a variety of practical reasons. Most clinicians have had little or minimal education about cannabis and cannabinoids. Also, most patients don't know what form of cannabis and what delivery method they will choose until they get to a dispensary. Usually, guidance on these aspects, as well as on the dose and titration methods, has been solely provided by the dispensary staff. The role of the clinician in the patient care process has been minimal. Even serious clinical matters, such as monitoring for efficacy, adverse effects, dependency, and possible diversion of the cannabis, have been relegated to variably trained dispensary staff members. In addition, the common practice of writing recommendation letters for a year's duration of medication has contributed a great deal to inadequate monitoring of patients using cannabis.

Once a patient has been determined to have a condition that may respond to medical cannabis and has been given a clinician's recommendation letter to take to the dispensary, clinician monitoring and follow-up visits are necessary. The recommendation letter should reflect the date by which the patient is expected to return for follow-up evaluation.

Before the patient leaves the clinician's office after the first visit, the provider should highlight the importance of starting out with a low dose and slowly increasing the dose or the frequency until an adequate clinical benefit is achieved or the adverse effects become unpleasant or disinhibiting.

The transient anxiety, paranoia, and tachycardia episodes sometimes associated with smoked or vaporized cannabis should be discussed, and the patient should be advised that these symptoms decrease dramatically with repeated use or with lower or less frequent doses.

The patient should be strongly advised that the psychoactive effects of the THC can impair driving, balance, and other cognitive and physical abilities. Therefore, cannabis should be used only in safe situations for the duration of these adverse effects of the medicine. At follow-up visits the clinician can discuss the psychoactive effects in more detail, as the patient will have become more familiar with how to avoid these effects through dosage titration, frequency, and routes of administration.

The clinician should, however, continue to recommend that the patient be diligent when using new cannabis products, since the psychoactive effects can vary considerably, even with the same cultivar of cannabis from the same dispensary.

As with any psychoactive medication, the clinician needs to be cognizant that the medication may be used by the patient for recreational purposes or diverted to other individuals. The patient should be made aware that this is illegal and will result in discontinuation of recommendation by the clinician. In general, urine drug testing for compliance is not helpful or recommended, however.

Of course, the patient should be told about other specific adverse effects that might indicate the need to prompt discontinuation of cannabis use, and to be advised to follow up earlier than scheduled if they occur.

Advising the Patient on Interaction with the Dispensary

When sending a patient to a dispensary for the first time, the clinician should advise him or her to have a detailed discussion with the dispensary staff. The discussion should include what cannabinoids or THC:CBD ratios are effective for the condition, the desirable percent of each cannabinoid, the type of cannabinoid product to use, and the routes of delivery. The patient should also learn how to calculate the dose and how to gradually titrate the dose upward.

After the patient has an understanding of these important details, he or she will usually purchase the delivery vehicle and a month's supply of cannabis, which is provided along with basic instructions by the dispensary, on how to use the delivery vehicle.

Basics of Clinician Monitoring

The next step is to determine appropriate monitoring and duration of time between follow-up visits. After the recommendation letter has been provided, the clinician and patient should agree on the date for an initial follow-up visit. This should be within two to four weeks, depending on the condition, the frequency of cannabis use, and need to evaluate whether another means of delivering the cannabis should be tried.

In addition, some clinicians may recommend that the patient purchase a hand-held cannabinoid analyzer. One popular brand is MyDx Analyzer (https://www.youtube.com/watch?v =G3P5nbQV7cU). These devices measure, fairly accurately, the percent of THC and CBD in the medical cannabis product. Newer versions may also calculate the amount of terpenes in the cannabis. These devices are very expensive, about $600, and are not generally necessary for medication monitoring; however, the technology is such that the price should drop dramatically in the coming years. Currently, this device is not covered by medical insurance. Patients will have to rely on the dispensary documentation about the THC and CBD content of cannabis plant material or on information provided on pre-packaged edibles. Patients should be reminded that the percentages or milligrams of THC and CBD documented by many dispensaries, and even on pre-packaged edibles, are notoriously wrong. Fortunately, the error is usually in over-estimating the percentages of both THC and CBD. For example, documentation for an edible item often states that there is more cannabinoid present than there actually is. Accurate knowledge of the THC and CBD content is very important to prevent adverse psychoactive effects and to ensure that the patient is actually getting a reasonable dose of the cannabinoids to be medically effective.

The clinician can advise the patient that there are several medical cannabis apps for smart phones and tablets, and more in development (http://appcrawlr.com/ios-apps/best-free-apps -marijuana). The patient can use these apps to track the usage, efficacy of the cannabis in treating symptoms, adverse effects, and different means of delivering cannabis. There is information on the website about local dispensaries and pricing of many of these apps.

PATIENT FOLLOW-UP

Monitoring a patient on medical cannabis is essentially the same as monitoring any other medication. The main differences are that there are a wide variety of forms that the drug comes in and a wide variety of means of delivering it, giving the clinician multiple ways to modify any side-effects and enhance therapeutic effects.

Medical cannabis can be recommended for a large variety of conditions but only after other more generally recognized treatment has been unsuccessful. Therefore, the main criterion for a clinician's recommending medical cannabis is how its benefits compare to those of previously used medications. Does the current regimen provide satisfactory relief? Is the cannabis likely to be superior to prior medications? Do the benefits of cannabis exceed the side-effects, logistical issues, costs, and other clinical issues?

MONITORING PSYCHOACTIVE EFFECTS OF THC

At the initial follow-up visit, the clinician should discuss the impact of the psychoactive effects of THC in the treatment regimen. Patients using cannabis regularly should start to notice a decrease in the adverse impact of its psychoactive effects after about two weeks of use. By the time of the first follow-up visit, the clinician should be able to identify how the beneficial effects and side-effects of the medication have changed.

During the time between the initial patient evaluation and the first follow-up visit, the patient will have gained experience in titrating the medication to get the best clinical impact and duration of effect. Learning to titrate, starting with low initial doses and slowly increasing doses or dosing frequency, is a vital component of what the patient needs to learn about using medical cannabis in the first few weeks.

At the initial follow-up visit, the clinician should discuss how the patient has modified titration of the cannabis as well as its efficacy, compared to other medications, current frequency of use, and adverse effects. If the patient has been using a medical cannabis app, the provider can look at a summary of the patient's documentation to help evaluate the medicine.

SCREENING FOR ADVERSE EFFECTS

At each follow-up visit, the clinician should screen the patient for early symptoms of psychological or physical dependence on cannabis. A variety of short written tests are available to monitor for developing dependence (https://ncpic.org.au/static/pdfs /background-papers/screening-and-assessment-for-cannabis -use-disorders.pdf). Most of these tests were designed for use with recreational users of cannabis and thus may not be appropriate for all patients. A team at Florida State University is developing a short, 5-minute screening test that the patient can complete at each visit, to help track the possible development of dependence. This test is called the *Medical Cannabis Dependence Tracking Questionnaire (MCDTQ)*. Other medical-cannabis specific apps in development will probably include a dependence-tracking component.

At the initial follow-up visit, the patient will no longer be naïve about the beneficial clinical effects, psychoactive effects, and side-effects of cannabis. If the medication is working better than previous medications, without the development of dependence or excessive adverse effects, then continuing cannabis is appropriate.

DOSING

If the cannabis has been medically beneficial but further benefit may be achieved, the provider should consider recommending a change in the dose or recommending a change in the frequency of use. If the onset of action or duration of action is not working for the patient, the type of cannabis product or means of delivery can be changed.

Based on what is determined as a result of each follow-up visit, the clinician needs to give the patient clear, documented instructions on the dose and frequency of use of the medication, as for any other medication. The patient can discuss these instructions in detail with dispensary staff members. Like other medications, especially addictive medications, the clinician should consider whether a refill or two is appropriate prior to re-evaluating the patient. If this is deemed appropriate, the clinician should provide the patient with a new recommendation letter, allowing the patient to continue to purchase restricted amounts of medical cannabis at a dispensary or, in some cases, to continue to grow cannabis plants.

> **Clinicians should never give a patient an automatic one-year recommendation.**

In the past, the clinician writing the recommendation letter often allowed for the use of medical cannabis for a year, prior to re-evaluating the patient. This is fraught with problems. The patient will have no compunction to be re-evaluated by the clinician for efficacy, side-effects, and the possible development of dependency. In addition, the clinician will lose his or her ability to interact with the patient because the patient will often perceive the dispensary staff, not the clinician, as the manager of the cannabis medication. In general, depending on the condition being treated and the pattern of use of cannabis, after the initial few visits help establish an effective dosing regimen, the clinician should re-evaluate the patient every six months, and, at each visit, a recommendation letter should be provided. The letter should cover the period of time before the next follow-up visit.

Other than the usual laboratory and diagnostic studies used to follow the medical condition, there are currently no specific diagnostic studies for ongoing cannabis use.

DRUG TESTING

If the clinician has a concern about possible diversion of the cannabis, a urine drug test for THC can be administered to the patient to confirm that he or she has used cannabis in the past few weeks to a month. However, this is ill advised. Most patients who might be diverting cannabis purchased at a dispensary often use a portion of it for themselves, usually recreationally, and sell the remainder.

Since cannabis has very few physiologic effects, there are no laboratory studies that will help the clinician better manage the patient. The crux of management revolves around evaluating the clinical efficacy compared to other treatments, minimizing the psychoactive effects, observing for the development of dependency or psychotic effects, and preventing accidental use by others, especially children. Patients using smoked cannabis need to be monitored for aggravation of pre-existing asthma or other airway disease.

CANNABIS DEPENDENCE
Cannabis dependence is associated with classic withdrawal symptoms, including anxiety, irritability, restlessness, insomnia, and poor appetite and other GI symptoms. These begin within hours to days of abstinence from cannabis, and resolve within a few weeks. It is not considered to be a serious medical condition. *See* Chapter 13 for more details.

An Uninsured Patient

A patient doesn't have insurance. After seeing you and being given a recommendation letter, he asks why you wrote the letter for only one month, not for a full year. He says his friend's doctor wrote one for a year, and he (your patient) can't afford to pay for frequent doctor's office visits. What can you tell him?

Discussion: You can tell him that many doctors are not comfortable with monitoring cannabis use or recommending changes to the cannabis regimen and route of administration. These doctors have left patient monitoring to the dispensary staff. However, you feel that clinicians should follow the patient using cannabis for its medicinal effects, the way any other medication would be monitored and managed. At the one-month follow-up visit, you can discuss the efficacy and side-effects of cannabis and perhaps recommend changes. In addition, at each visit you will be monitoring the patient for psychological and physical dependence, which occurs in up to 10 percent of cannabis users.

You can tell him, usually after the first follow-up visit, that he won't need to be seen for six months.

CHAPTER 13

Cannabis Dependence and Psychological Adverse Effects

There has long been controversy over whether regular cannabis users become addicted. The literature clearly shows that about 9 percent of adult recreational users develop psychological dependence, with classic tolerance and withdrawal symptoms. The rate of cannabis withdrawal is higher, 10–20 percent, in persons who use cannabis daily. The Diagnostic and Statistical Manual of Mental Disorders (DSM-5) describes cannabis dependence (ICD-9 394.3) as a condition marked by irritability, nervousness, sleep difficulty, decreased appetite, depressed mood, and physical symptoms of discomfort.[124]

Most patients with cannabis dependence syndrome can be treated on an out-patient basis. There is a high proportion of comorbid psychological or psychiatric conditions among persons seeking treatment for cannabis dependence. Persons seeking treatment for cannabis dependence average 10 years of near-daily use and more than six failed attempts to quit.[124]

The syndrome is marked by the development of tolerance and withdrawal symptoms. By definition, it includes continued use of the drug despite social, legal, psychological, and physical adverse consequences. The number of rehabilitation admissions for cannabis dependence treatment is increasing exponentially in recent years.

Unlike physical ailments and cannabis use, there is quite a large body of scientific data about cannabis and mental health issues.

The same mental health and socioeconomic factors associated with alcohol and other drug dependence are associated with cannabis dependence.[125-127] Cannabis is the most commonly identified illicit substance used by people admitted to drug rehabilitation programs for dependency. There may be some confounding because many cannabis users start using it to treat pre-existing symptoms such as anxiety or for mood elevation.

Risk Factors for Cannabis Dependence

As discussed in Chapter 10 on pharmacogenetic testing, certain genetic phenotypes have a predisposition to becoming dependent.

In addition to the negative effects of cannabis on neural development and cognitive function in adolescents, being of a young age at the time when cannabis use is first started is also associated with psychological dependence.[128]

Frequent and heavy use of cannabis is associated with symptoms of dependence. Prolonged use of cannabis has been shown to have both pharmacodynamic and pharmacokinetic effects that require higher doses of the drug to achieve the same effect. In addition, long-term users of cannabis become tolerant to the psychoactive effects of THC via changes in the cannabinoid receptor function in the brain and body.

The clinician recommending cannabis for medical therapy should remain both cognizant and vigilant for escalating dosing of THC, and onset of dependence symptoms between doses.

Treatment of Cannabis Dependence

Symptoms of withdrawal are usually not as severe as with those of withdrawal from other drugs. Symptoms include the onset of anger, dysphoria, disturbed sleep patterns, and loss of appetite, starting within hours to a day after discontinuing the use of cannabis. There is no specific medication that alleviates withdrawal symptoms; psychological counseling is all that can be offered. Most symptoms resolve within a few weeks of abstinence.

One case report suggested that CBD, alone, can be used to reduce the anxiety associated with cannabis withdrawal.[129] Additional studies are needed.

Screen for Risk of Dependence Syndrome

It is important that patients requesting cannabis therapy be thoroughly evaluated by the clinician for increased risk of developing dependence syndrome. Prior dependence syndromes with cannabis or other substances, family history of dependence syndromes, adolescent age at onset, and other socioeconomic factors are well-known risk factors for developing cannabis dependence syndrome.

Several quick and easy-to-use self-report questionnaires and physician-directed questionnaires are readily available. Different screening tests should be used for adolescent patients and adults. There are tools that can be used by the clinician prior to initiating cannabis therapy and other tools to use at regularly scheduled follow-up visits to help identify, early on, the development of cannabis dependence. The National Cannabis Prevention and Information Centre has an informative description and list of simple self-reporting screening tools that are currently available. Self-reporting is felt to be generally reliable and valid across various types of patients. (https://ncpic.org.au /static/pdfs/background-papers/screening-and-assessment-for -cannabis-use-disorders.pdf)

Most of the symptoms and conditions for which cannabis therapy may be effective can be treated with other medications that do not cause dependence syndrome. Therefore, prior to initiating or continuing cannabis therapy, the clinician should be confident that the patient is not one of the 9 percent likely to develop cannabis dependence syndrome.

Patients who develop a significant cannabis dependence syndrome should be considered for referral to a drug treatment program.

Screening for Adverse Psychological and Psychiatric Effects

There has long been an association between cannabis use and various psychological conditions or symptoms.[130] There are literally hundreds of articles in the literature regarding adverse psychological responses to cannabis use. Generally, these fall into two main categories: (1) acute, self-limited dose-response conditions and (2) chronic psychiatric conditions. Acute conditions such as anxiety, agitation, and psychosis are generally in response to excessive intake of THC. Most of these temporary dose-related symptoms can be mitigated by also decreasing the frequency of dosing or concentration of THC. Low doses of THC tend to be anxiolytic, whereas higher blood concentrations tend to produce anxiety.[131]

Separately, a review of several studies has concluded that adverse psychological and psychoactive effects can be mitigated by the concomitant presence of CBD by means of the entourage effect.[132]

DEPERSONALIZATION

Depersonalization is a state in which one's thoughts and feelings seem unreal and not to belong to oneself, or where one loses one's sense of identity. This is a temporary and self-limited symptom that has long been recognized in those who use cannabis excessively; it may be due to neurotoxicity from cannabis metabolites.[133]

DEPRESSION

Users of cannabis have long noted it to be a temporary mood elevator.

Research in animal models and human studies has confirmed that THC may be useful in treating depression caused by chronic stress. Chronic stress reduces the production of the naturally occurring endocannabinoids. Using THC increases endocannabinoid function on CB1 receptors within the brain, stabilizing mood and easing stress-related depression.

However, many studies suggest that long-term use of cannabis increases the risk for depression,[134] suicidal ideation,[135] and suicide.[136]

Regular use in adolescents is possibly a risk for depression, anxiety,[137] and bipolar disorder[138] later in life. However, because of the confounding issues of pre-existing symptoms in adolescents and onset of cannabis use, the studies are inconclusive about causation.

Previous studies have been inconclusive about the effect of cannabis on dopamine levels. However, the Brookhaven National Laboratory recently conducted a study of 24 persons who had been smoking several times a day for many years and 24 control subjects.[139] They found a blunted response to dopamine release in the habitual smokers, compared to the control group. It is not clear if habitual smokers had pre-existing negative moods and were more prone to self-medicate, or if the blunted response was a consequence of prolonged cannabis use. The study concluded that it was possible that prolonged, regular use of cannabis use may increase depression and anxiety. The investigators also felt that excessive cannabis use may damage the brain's reward circuitry.

Clinicians should be aware of the onset of depression associated with chronic use of cannabis. Simple self-report screening tools can be combined with other screening methodologies as part of follow-up visits.

ANXIETY

The relationship between cannabis use and anxiety is complex and often contradictory. While most persons using cannabis associate it with a calming, mood-elevating effect, a significant portion of users have occasional anxiety episodes. Some of the anxiety effects are due to the sympathomimetic effects on heart rate, lightheadedness due to hypotension, or feelings of depersonalization.

Frequent cannabis users have been repeatedly shown to have a high prevalence of anxiety disorder; likewise, individuals with anxiety disorders have relatively high rates of cannabis use. This confounding effect has made it difficult to determine if cannabis causes chronic anxiety disorders.[140]

However, as discussed previously, many persons have an acute, self-limited anxiety reaction or even a panic episode in response to higher levels of THC, especially when the THC is not counter-balanced with CBD. Balancing THC with CBD has been shown to reduce acute anxiety symptoms by 50 percent.[3,17]

Since most of the available anxiolytic pharmaceuticals have significant safety issues, and more severe dependency issues, using cannabis for the treatment of anxiety disorders may be appropriate in carefully screened and selected patients. A balanced cannabis medication with a 1:1 ratio of CBD:THC, and a low to medium percentage of THC, is recommended when treating anxiety symptoms or when someone has a history of anxiety.

PSYCHOSIS OR SCHIZOPHRENIA

Cannabis, more specifically THC, has long been associated with acute and transient psychosis in otherwise healthy persons. Many studies have also shown that early and heavy cannabis use is associated with psychosis that resembles schizophrenia later in life.[141-144] High-THC cannabis is particularly associated with psychosis. However, chronic cannabis-related psychosis usually resolves with discontinuance of the cannabis. There is evidence of a genetic predisposition toward cannabis-related psychosis and schizophrenia.[36,37,145] Again, there are confounding factors when it comes to clarifying causation issues.

There is evidence that THC can worsen previously stable psychotic disorders and may trigger a chronic psychotic disorder in individuals with a family history of psychosis.

The synthetic THC analogues found in "herbal incense" designer drugs carry a particularly high risk for precipitating psychotic episodes.

There are several short and simple screening tools for clinicians to use to assess family history and risk for future development of psychosis and schizophrenia. In general, persons at increased risk for development of psychosis or schizophrenia should not be treated with medium- or high-THC cannabis.

CHAPTER 14

Specific Types of Patients and Related Issues

At this time, patients who are going to be using medical cannabis may be different in several ways from the typical patient who will comfortably take medications from a local drug store. This chapter provides a general discussion of the various types of patients and issues that can arise when starting a patient on medical cannabis.

Veteran Patients

The most common type of patient presenting for a recommendation of medical cannabis is an adult who has had prior experience with recreational cannabis and has noticed that it helps with a chronic pain condition, anxiety, or insomnia. Or, the person may tell the clinician that a friend with a similar problem does well with medical cannabis. I call these patients *veteran patients*. In many respects, not only are they the majority of patients, but they also are the easiest to manage medically.

These patients are usually not naïve or unfamiliar with the psychoactive effects of THC or the side-effects of dry mouth, temporary elevated levels of anxiety, bloodshot eyes, palpitations, or the possibility of transient paranoia. In fact, if they are recreational cannabis users, they probably are already somewhat inured to the side-effects. With this type of patient, the main issue that the clinician needs to consider is that they could be seeking a recommendation letter in order to obtain cannabis merely for recreational purposes, without any true medical need.

As for all patients being started on medical cannabis, the clinician needs to obtain a history of the condition, discuss whether the patient has previously tried other more generally recognized treatments, and ask why the patient feels that adding medical cannabis should be the next step in treatment. A thorough evaluation of this type of patient should successfully screen out drug-seekers and prevent diversion of medical cannabis to recreational uses.

Because this type of patient is not naïve to the effects of cannabis, he or she will usually already be familiar with titrating the dose of the medication, the difference in onset and duration of action of the various forms of cannabis, and the different delivery vehicles.

With these veteran patients, at each follow-up visit the clinician should remain cognizant of possible physical or psychological dependence or diversion of the medication for recreational use or sale to others.

Naïve Patients

The next type of patient is one who has never used cannabis before, or at least not regularly, and who, after reading about it or talking to friends about it, wanted to try it for management of a chronic medical condition. I call these *naïve patients*. These patients generally have a more clearly identifiable need for medical cannabis and are unhappy with the efficacy or side-effects from other medications. The clinician may conclude that all of the generally recognized treatments have, in fact, been ineffective and recommend adding medical cannabis.

Again, the clinician needs to take a detailed medical history to make certain that the more generally-recognized treatments have been maximized and that all of the available standard treatments have been tried.

The most difficult issue with naïve patients is preparing them for the psychoactive effects of the cannabis, especially higher-THC cannabis. The clinician needs to provide detailed education about the various psychoactive effects and warn the patient about the hazards of operating vehicles, dangerous machinery, and similar issues while taking medical cannabis. The concept of titrating doses is likely to be new to these patients, so reminding them to start at a low dose and slowly titrate up, is vital to reducing untoward side-effects and maintaining compliance with the treatment plan.

The clinician will also need to impress upon the patient the fact that most of the medical effects occur at lower blood concentrations of the cannabinoids than do the psychoactive effects. So, the onset of psychoactive effects is a signal that they have more than enough cannabinoids working in their blood stream.

Salvage Patients

This general patient category includes a very limited number of patients with chronic conditions for which medical cannabis may be effective and should be recommended, even if the patient is initially adverse to using cannabis.

These conditions are rare and are usually handled by sub-specialists. They include Dravet seizures (approximately 5,000 cases in the U.S.), Lennox-Gastaut syndrome (approximately 15,000 cases in the U.S.), severe, intractable CINV, and a few other rare conditions.

Pregnant Patients

Pregnant women may ask their primary care provider about using cannabis during pregnancy. They may be habitual cannabis users and want to know if continued use will harm the fetus, or they may want to try to get relief from nausea and other pregnancy-related symptoms. Cannabis is the most commonly used illicit substance among pregnant women. National self-report studies show that 2–6 percent of pregnant women aged 18–25 have used cannabis in the month prior to the survey. A British study found that cannabis was the only illicit drug pregnant women were likely to continue using to term.

There is a handful of animal and epidemiologic studies regarding the use of prenatal use of cannabis.[146–148] Cannabinoids rapidly cross the placental barrier and enter the fetus. The studies suggest an association with decreased birth weight and negative effects on the developing brain, namely, increased irritability and arousal in the first few days after birth and both learning disabilities and memory impairment later in infancy and early childhood. Heavy use of cannabis prenatally and use during pregnancy were associated with more cognitive and short-term memory issues.

In past decades, *in vitro* and *in vivo* animal studies suggested the possibility of teratogenic and mutagenic effects related to cannabis, but this has not been borne out by more recent studies.

For the reasons described above, pregnant women should be strongly cautioned against using cannabis during pregnancy or while attempting to become pregnant.

Breastfeeding Women

Like pregnant women, many breastfeeding women are regular users of cannabis and may feel that there is a medicinal value to their infant from using cannabis while breastfeeding. Ingested or inhaled cannabinoids are rapidly transferred into breast milk. Higher or more frequent doses of cannabis are associated with higher levels in breast milk and more long-term storage of the cannabinoids in the body fat. Infants who have been breastfed by women who use cannabis can have positive urine test results for THC for up to three weeks after ingesting the breast milk. However, the amount of THC transferred via the breast milk is not enough to cause psychoactive effects.

There are few studies on the effects on the infant of using cannabis while breastfeeding; however, the American Academy of Pediatrics strongly discourages the use of cannabis while breastfeeding because of concerns about infant brain development.[149]

There is an informative review on the Canadian Family Physician website (www.cfp.ca/content/51/3/349.full.pdf) titled "Marijuana Use and Breastfeeding."

Opioid-Dependent Patients

Cannabis can be used very effectively to help reduce the dose of opioid medications or to help transition a patient off opioids to non-opioid pain relievers. Persons with a prior history of drug dependence are at increased risk for cannabis dependence syndrome. In addition, the psychoactive effects of opioids and the common use of benzodiazepines make adverse psychoactive effects from the use of cannabis much more likely. This is discussed in detail in Chapter 13.

This group of patients would also be at much higher risk for using cannabis recreationally or possibly for diversion of the cannabis to others. These patients require close and very regular monitoring of the use of cannabis and other medications.

Psychotic Patients

About 1 in 10 patients experience temporary psychosis from use of cannabis. This is discussed in greater detail in Chapter 13. Psychosis has been shown to be more likely in patients using high-potency-THC cannabis. Persons with a prior history or family history of psychosis or schizophrenia are at much greater risk for psychosis from cannabis use.[136,150] The benefits should outweigh the risks of adding cannabis to the treatment regimen, and the patient should be closely and regularly monitored for temporary symptoms of psychosis.

Patients with Prior Drug Dependence

Patients with a prior history of drug dependence, whether the drug was prescribed or illicit, are at increased risk for developing cannabis dependence syndrome. This is discussed in detail in Chapter 13. On average, about 1 in 10 patients develop cannabis dependence syndrome; however, it may be twice this level in patients with a prior history of drug dependence.

As with opioid patients, this group of patients are much more likely to use cannabis recreationally or to divert the cannabis to others. These patients require close and very regular monitoring of both cannabis use and the use of other medications.[35,128]

Adolescents and Children

Except for the use of very low-THC, high-CBD cannabis for severe childhood epilepsy syndromes, cannabis is not recommended for children and adolescents. This is discussed in more detail in Chapter 9. Adolescents are prone to increased safety risks when, for example, operating vehicles or bicycles. There is also increased risk for long term-cognitive issues, dependency, and adverse effects in adolescents and children.[151,152]

Elderly Patients

Elderly patients are at increased risk for pre-existing cognitive deficits, problems with balance, and adverse effects from the psychoactive effects of THC. In addition, the concept of titration of dose and the complexity of administering and timing cannabis medications are often more challenging in elderly patients. Each patient should be evaluated for how appropriate cannabis medication would be as an adjunct therapy.

Patients Working in Hazardous Environments

Patients who have occupations or hobbies that place them in hazardous environments or conditions should be evaluated for appropriateness of cannabis medication. Especially early on in treatment, the psychoactive effects of the THC can greatly increase the hazards in the environment. Other performance issues may occur as a result of the psychoactive effects of THC.

Palliative Care Patients

Patients undergoing palliative care are probably the most impacted by appropriate use of cannabis medication. The many positive effects of cannabis on pain, inflammation, nausea, appetite, and mood are particularly noticeable in palliative care patients. However, the cognitive deficits, age, concomitant medications, and other impairments associated with palliative care patients make maximizing therapeutic efficacy challenging.

CHAPTER 15

Insurance and Coding Issues

his is the shortest chapter in the text because, for the most part, there is no difference between health insurance reimbursement for conditions treated with medical cannabis and all other medical conditions. Cannabis will be only an adjunct to the other medications and therapy that the patient is already receiving for the condition.

As far as coding is concerned, there is only one additional code to use when recommending medical cannabis as part of a treatment plan, unless the patient develops side-effects or cannabis-dependence syndrome, in which case coding for these conditions can be included.

When billing the health insurance company for the evaluation and management of a patient, the fact that the patient is using medical cannabis as part of their treatment is irrelevant. The insurance company reimburses the clinician for the evaluation and management of the conditions, symptoms, or specific diagnosis. In addition, any diagnostic testing done for medical evaluation is covered, whether or not the clinician is recommending cannabis.

Pharmacogenetic Testing

The only special circumstance would be if pharmacogenetic testing is done, as discussed in Chapter 10. This testing can be used to assist in reducing the risk of cannabis dependence, dosing of THC, or prevention of psychotic breaks from THC. Pharmacogenetic testing is a burgeoning area, and it's use has been determined to be medically necessary for some drugs in some patient populations. Some examples of drugs include clopido-grel, tetrabenazine, and eliglustat. Testing for specific geno-typing and mutations are reimbursable for these very specific clinical scenarios. Pharmacogenetic testing is being recommended for an ever-increasing number of drugs as part of the trend toward personalized medicine, based on genetic profiles, a rapidly expanding clinical frontier.

However, pharmacogenetic testing is currently still in its infancy and, for the most part, health insurance companies would consider pharmacogenetic testing prior to using THC based medication as "experimental or investigational" and would not cover the testing. Nonetheless, it is expected that, in the near future, pharmacogenetic testing will become more applicable for evaluating patients at increased risk for psychosis and for dependency syndromes from cannabinoid use. The pre-certification process will vary by insurance company, and the allowable conditions or ICD codes will vary as well.

The cost of cannabis and paraphernalia is not a covered expense.

The actual cannabis and paraphernalia necessary to administer cannabis is currently not a covered expense and probably won't ever be covered. Health insurance companies pay only for medically necessary FDA-approved drugs. Even if, as is expected very soon, cannabis is moved from Schedule I to Schedule II or III, the cannabis plant material (flower bud, extracted oil, or edibles made from these) will not be an FDA-approved medica-tion, so the patient will probably need to continue to pay for these expenses.

However, FDA-approved cannabis medications, such as possibly Sativex, may be a covered medical expense for certain medical conditions and become available at pharmacies.

Coding

When a patient is started on medical cannabis, the following V-code, ICD-9-CM V58.69, is recommended. This is for "long-term (current) use of other medication." The ICD-10-CM conver-sion would be Z79.899, "other long-term (current) drug therapy." The cannabis is not specifically identified with either code.

There is a wide array of ICD9 and ICD10 codes for cannabis-related conditions, such as drug dependence syndrome, psychological side-effects, and cannabinoid hyperemesis syndrome.

Working with Other Professionals in the Community

M edical cannabis has been legal in some states for almost two decades. A pattern of medical practice has developed in which a tiny portion of the clinicians in a community see most of the patients who are using medical cannabis. This is not unlike how pain management clinics have burgeoned over the past decade, with most opioids and long-term benzodiazepines now being prescribed to patients at these clinics. At the same time, these patients maintain a separate relationship with their primary care clinician for prescription of their other medications and conditions.

There are probably a number of reasons for this current situation with medical cannabis clinicians. There is still a social stigma attached to cannabis use, although in the past few years this has been disappearing in many areas. Many clinicians do not want to be associated with what was, and still is in many states, an illegal drug. There is the issue of the type of patients who want to use cannabis as medicine. The clinician may view patients who request a recommendation for use of medical cannabis as drug seekers (recreational users), trying to get cannabis for recreational purposes. Or they may see these patients as potentially getting the cannabis to sell and divert it to others for recreational use, as has occurred with opiates and "pill mills" around the country.

Also, there is the fact that most patients who are treated with cannabis have either chronic pain or anxiety-related conditions, and a clinician may not be comfortable treating these conditions, with or without cannabis. Finally, in the past, the conditions treated with cannabis and cannabinoid pharmaceuticals have been limited to chemo-induced nausea and vomiting (CINV), and HIV-associated cachexia, and the clinician may not see these types of patients.

However, the biggest reason for the clinical separation of clinicians who recommend medical cannabis from the rest of the medical community may be a lack of education and practical clinical experience in most clinicians. A survey conducted by this author of United States and Canadian medical and osteopathic schools found that only a small portion offer any kind of formal or required training on the subject. A small portion were considering adding one to four hours of training in future curricula. In addition, almost all of the textbooks that discuss medical cannabis are folksy or anecdotal in nature, without sound, evidence-based discussion or a critical analysis of the topic.

When a clinician has acquired the knowledge provided in this book, and continues to learn from other sources and patient experience afterward, they are much more likely to start regularly considering adding cannabis as an adjunct medication to their arma. This is especially true in the future, when patients of all ages and from various cultural and socioeconomic groups will be asking if cannabis may be helpful for their condition.

Referral to Another Clinician

For the time being, if a clinician is currently recommending cannabis for a patient and needs to refer the patient to a specialist for another condition, the clinician will have to communicate some essential information about the cannabis treatment to the other clinician.

In the future, as the use of medical cannabis becomes *de rigueur*, it can be expected that the other clinicians will have an understanding of how cannabis works and what patient monitoring should be done to identify drug-drug interactions, side-effects, and other effects of the medication.

Currently, it is recommended that when referring a patient who is using medical cannabis to another clinician, a standard statement be included in the referral letter, stating the patient's use of cannabis, for what conditions, how much, and by what means. The following is an example of such a statement:

> *"Miss Smith has been followed by me for the past year for chronic insomnia. She had trouble with standard pharmaceuticals for insomnia and was started on medical cannabis six months ago. She has responded well to the use of bedtime medical cannabis. Most nights, she smokes approximately a ½-gm cannabis cigarette shortly before bedtime, for the immediate drowsiness that it causes. She shows no evidence of dependence or escalation of use of the cannabis. She denies recreational use of the medicine. If I can provide additional information, please do not hesitate to contact me."*

LOCAL RESOURCE FOR OTHER CLINICIANS

It is likely that a clinician who regularly recommends medical cannabis in his practice may garner a reputation among other clinicians in the community. It is not unexpected that community clinicians will be referring or recommending their patients to this clinician, especially if they are uncomfortable or inexperienced in the subject or have questions about using medical cannabis for a condition or symptom. In this scenario, the clinician should not expect a letter from the referring clinician. Most of the time, the clinician in the community will know that a particular provider recommends medical cannabis regularly with his patients and will suggest to the patient that he or she contact the clinician directly to discuss cannabis treatment. Often, the patient will continue to obtain the generally recommended medications from the original clinician, and the other clinician will follow the patient only for the use of the cannabis.

In states where medical cannabis has been legal for some time, a small group of clinicians has given medical cannabis a bad reputation. These clinicians will often have gaudy advertising and promotional materials, and essentially guarantee that any person presenting to their clinic will be given a recommendation letter and Medical Cannabis Card for a cash fee. Usually, these clinicians do only a screening history and a cursory examination prior to writing the recommendation letter. There are several clinicians who do the consultation via a computer or tablet device. Usually, they will make the recommendation good for a year's supply of cannabis and provide minimal advice, counseling, and follow-up to their patients. It is expected that this "Wild West" attitude toward medical cannabis will gradually disappear as the benefits and efficacy of medical cannabis become well appreciated by the entire medical community.

It is expected that in the future medical cannabis will become an accepted therapeutic option in primary care practice and that using medical cannabis for the wide variety of conditions for which it is helpful will not become some sort of ill-defined specialty or isolated clinical practice.

CLINICAL SCENARIO
Referral of Patient to Another Clinician

You have a patient on infrequent doses of medical cannabis for episodic anxiety. She needs to be referred to a gynecologist for menstrual issues. What should you tell the gynecologist in your referral note?

Discussion: Medical cannabis is still widely considered unacceptable as a therapeutic agent, and most clinicians are not comfortable with how it works or how it interacts with other medications. Even in states where medical cannabis has been legal for well over a decade, 90 percent of doctors have not recommended it for their patients.

Given this scenario, it is appropriate, for the clinician, when referring a patient to another physician, to document the fact that the patient is using cannabis as recommended therapy. How frequently it is used and how it is administered should be described. You can mention that, in general, cannabis does not interact with most pharmaceuticals when it is used only intermittently, as in this patient.

Medical Caregivers

The original concept behind the legislation for medical cannabis was that it would be used only for severe, chronic, and debilitating diseases or conditions. It was expected that the patients would have already had maximum therapy with generally accepted medications and were still symptomatic.

All the state initiatives or legislation recognized that because patients using cannabis would be chronically debilitated, they would allow for registered medical caregivers. The caregivers are generally defined as individuals or organizations who can possess, cultivate, and provide medical cannabis to qualified medical cannabis patients. The rules vary by state, but in general they have to be either over 18 or 21 years of age, not be a felon, and be registered with the state to be the caregiver to the specific patient. They are generally allowed to care for one to five patients, depending on the state. No specific training is required. Like the patients, there is usually a registry of these individuals.

For very sick or debilitated patients, caregivers provide the patient with cannabis, along with necessary supplies, at regular intervals. The caregiver can either cultivate the necessary cannabis or obtain it at a dispensary.

There are usually generally recognized fees for these services; these fees are not reimbursed by health insurance.

The patient will then have to go to the clinician to be evaluated and obtain a recommendation letter for the next period of treatment. But once this is obtained, the caregiver can then get the next batch of medical cannabis and provide it to the patient for the duration of time documented on the recommendation letter.

Each state that has legalized medical cannabis has independently run websites. These provide information on how to find a medical caregiver. In addition, there is a national website, www.marijuana-caregiver.com, that provides this service for each state as well as other helpful information about caregivers to patients.

Dispensary Staff

Currently, there are no officially recognized training courses, websites, or materials for dispensary staff. However, there is a growing number of serious academic medical cannabis establishments around the country—Medical Marijuana United, Oaksterdam University in California, and Cannabis University Inc. of Colorado, to name a few. These institutions provide training on cultivation of cannabis plants and separately provide training courses to dispensary staff. Graduates of these short programs usually have a basic knowledge, to varying degrees, about cultivars of cannabis, edibles, and tinctures. They can recommend which of these might be best for a particular patient's specific symptoms. The graduates are also trained to determine the percentage of THC and CBD in the plant materials so they can help patients with dosing and side-effects. They also can recommend the best route of administration. Prior to complying with the physician's recommendation, some of the more experienced dispensary staff members will consider the patient's age, co-morbid medical conditions, medications, severity of symptoms, and experience with prior cannabis use. However, most staff will only have a cursory understanding of the disease or condition and will focus more on symptom relief, dosing, and gradual titration of the cannabinoids.

Dispensaries have a wide variety of supplies and paraphernalia used to administer the cannabis. They usually have manufactured edible products and home-made edibles as well.

Health insurance companies do not pay for non-FDA-approved medications. For this reason, even though the doctor's visits, laboratory testing, and other medical expenses are generally covered, the actual cannabis, necessary paraphernalia, and caregiver fee are not. Because of this, the patient or caregiver going to a cannabis dispensary will have to pay for the cannabis and any paraphernalia out of pocket. In fact, payment in cash will probably be necessary because, even though medical cannabis is legal at a state level, the banking rules are federal, and cannabis sales are illegal under federal banking rules. This situation will be remedied if cannabis is changed from Schedule I to Schedule II or III or if the proposed federal banking rule amendments are implemented.

Once the patient has been evaluated by the clinician and the recommendation letter provided, the patient or caretaker takes the letter to a local dispensary. There, the staff enters the patient into the state medical marijuana registry and gets the patient a Medical Cannabis Card. The actual logistics vary by state. The clinician has historically taken a supervisory role. The dispensary staff and caregiver, if the patient has one, maintain a close working relationship in recommending changes in dosing, cultivars of cannabis, and routes of administration. The clinician traditionally has the patient return for an initial follow-up visit within 2–4 weeks to check for efficacy, side-effects, compliance, and possible dependence. Much like the clinical management of other chronic but stable diseases, this is often followed by semi-annual monitoring and re-assessment visits.

The Role of the Dispensary and the Clinician's Role

The dispensary staff is often very helpful with picking specific strains of cannabis for their potency and THC:CBD ratio. They also can be helpful with more logistical and pragmatic issues related to dosing, titrating, and using the medication in different scenarios. However, in addition to monitoring for efficacy and adverse effects, the clinician needs to take the supervisory role in directing the patient and dispensary staff as to the desired onset and duration of action.

That being said, the clinician should understand that there is very little training, standardization, or certification of the staff members at these dispensaries. Therefore, the clinician must be aware of how this reality can affect clinical outcomes of patients using cannabis. This unfortunate training and certification situation should change in the future.

| *The clinician should keep at arm's length from the dispensary.*

In order to comply with federal, state and insurance law, clinicians need to keep at arm's length from any association or affiliation with, or financial incentives from, the independent cannabis dispensaries. They may receive training and educational materials for use in their practice from the dispensaries. However, liaison and regular communication between the clinician and dispensary staff is recommended. This is for logistical and organizational purposes and to prevent diversion.

It is recommended that the clinician visit some of the local dispensaries to become familiar with the types of paraphernalia for delivery of the medicine and what kind of edibles are available. He or she can also get a sense of how educated and experienced the staff are, and at the same time, open lines of communication with the staff to better help patients and caregivers.

CLINICAL SCENARIO

Patient's Request for Recommendation of a Dispensary

You have just written a recommendation letter for a patient to start cannabis therapy. She asks if you can recommend a dispensary. She asks if you work closely with any dispensary. What can you tell her?

Discussion: It is imperative that the physician remain at arms' length from dispensaries in matters of business or finance. However, the physician can and should be aware of the quality, service, products, and relative pricing of the local dispensaries. Open communication and ongoing professional interaction with local dispensaries is highly recommended. Therefore, if the physician has familiarity with dispensaries, he or she can recommend one, especially one with which he or she is very familiar.

References

1. Khey DN, Stogner J, Miller BL. *Emerging drugs, today versus yesteryear. Emerging Trends in Drug Use and Distribution*. Springer Briefs in Criminology, 2014;12:13–32.
2. Borgelt LM, Franson KL, Nussbaum AM, et al. The pharmacologic and clinical effects of medical cannabis. *Pharmacotherapy* 2013; 33:195–209.
3. Karniol IG, Shirakawa I, Kasinski N, et al. Cannabidiol interferes with the effects of delta 9-tetrahydrocannabinol in man. *Eur J Pharmacol* 1974;28:172–177.
4. Hemp Industries Association USA LLC v. Drug Enforcement Administration, nos. 03-71366, 03-71693. US 9th Circuit. February 6, 2004. Available at: http://caselaw.findlaw.com/us-9th-circuit /1253723.html. Accessed January 28, 2015.
5. Cunha JM, Carlini EA, Pereira AE, et al. Chronic administration of cannabidiol to healthy volunteers and epileptic patients. *Pharmacology* 1980;21:175–185.
6. Zuardi AW, Hallak JE, Dursun SM, et al. Cannabidiol monotherapy for treatment resistant schizophrenia. *J Psychopharmacol* 2006; 20:683–686.
7. Zuardi AW, Crippa J, Dursun S, et al. Cannabidiol was ineffective for manic episode of bipolar affective disorder. *J Psychopharmacol* 2010;24:135–137.
8. Mincis M, Pfeferman A, Guimaraes RX, et al. Chronic administration of cannabidiol in man: pilot study. *AMB Rev Assoc Med Bras* 1973; 19:185–190.
9. Zuardi AW, Crippa J, Hallak J, et al. Cannabidiol for the treatment of psychosis in Parkinson's disease. *J Psychopharmacol* 2009; 23:979–983.
10. Zuardi AW, Guimaraes FS, Moreira AC. Effect of cannabidiol on plasma prolactin, growth hormone and cortisol in human volunteers. *Braz J Med Biol Res* 1993;26:213–217.
11. Zhornitsky S, Potvin S. Cannabidiol in humans-the quest for therapeutic targets. *Pharmaceuticals (Basel)* 2012;5:529–552.

12. Bergamaschi MM, Queiroz RH, Zuardi AW, et al. Safety and side effects of cannabidiol, a Cannabis sativa constituent. *Curr Drug Saf* 2011;6:237–249.

13. Morgan CJ, Curran HV. Effects of cannabidiol on schizophrenia-like symptoms in people who use cannabis. *Br J Psychiatry* 2008;192:306–307.

14. Morgan CJ, Schafer G, Freeman TP, et al. Impact of cannabidiol on the acute memory and psychotomimetic effects of smoked cannabis: naturalistic study [corrected]. *Br J Psychiatry* 2010; 197:285–290.

15. Bhattacharyya S, Morrison PD, Fusar-Poli P, et al. Opposite effects of delta-9-tetrahydrocannabinol and cannabidiol on human brain function and psychopathology. *Neuropsychopharmacology* 2010; 35:764–774.

16. Schubart CD, Sommer IE, van Gastel WA, et al. Cannabis with high cannabidiol content is associated with fewer psychotic experiences. *Schizophr Res* 2011;130:216–221.

17. Dalton WS, Martz R, Lemberger L, et al. Influence of cannabidiol on delta-9-tetrahydrocannabinol effects. *Clin Pharmacol Ther* 1976; 19:300–309.

18. Deiana S, Watanabe A, Yamasaki Y, et al. Plasma and brain pharmacokinetic profile of cannabidiol (CBD), cannabidivarine (CBDV), delta-9-tetrahydrocannabivarin (THCV,) and cannabigerol (CBG) in rats and mice following oral and intraperitoneal administration and CBD action on obsessive-compulsive behavior. *Psychopharmacology (Berl)* 2012;219:859–873.

19. Hawksworth G, McArdle K. *Metabolism and Pharmacokinetics of Cannabinoids.* London: Pharmaceutical Press, 2004.

20. Paudel KS, Hammel DC, Agu RU, et al. Cannabidiol bioavailability after nasal and transdermal application: effect of permeation enhancers. *Drug Dev Ind Pharm* 2010;36:1088–1097.

21. Solowij N, Broyd SJ, van Hell HH, et al. A protocol for the delivery of cannabidiol (CBD) and combined CBD and 9-tetrahydrocannabinol (THC) by vaporisation. *BMC Pharmacol Toxicol* 2014;15:58.

22. Welty TE, Luebke A, Gidal BE. Cannabidiol: promise and pitfalls. *Epilepsy Curr* 2014;14:250–252.

23. Sznitman SR, Zolotov Y. Cannabis for therapeutic purposes and public health and safety: a systematic and critical review. *Int J Drug Policy* 2015;26:20–29.

24. Crean RD, Crane NA, Mason BJ. An evidence-based review of acute and long-term effects of cannabis use on executive cognitive functions. *J Addict Med* 2011;5:1–8.

25. Meier MH, Caspi A, Ambler A, et al. Persistent cannabis users show neuropsychological decline from childhood to midlife. *Proc Natl Acad Sci USA* 2012;109:E2657–E2664.

26. Solowij N, Yucel M, Lorenzetti V, et al. Does cannabis cause lasting brain damage? In: Castle D, Murray RM, D'Souza DC, eds. Cambridge, UK: Cambridge University Press; 2012:103–113.

27. Chen J, McCarron RM. Cannabinoid hyperemesis syndrome: a result of chronic, heavy cannabis use. *Current Psychiatr* 2013; 12:48–54.

28. Karschner EL, Darwin WD, Goodwin RS, et al. Plasma cannabinoid pharmacokinetics following controlled oral delta-9-tetrahydrocannabinol and oromucosal cannabis extract administration. *Clin Chem* 2011;57:66–75.

29. Elkashef A, Vocci F, Huestis M. Marijuana neurobiology and treatment. *Subst Abus* 2008; 29(3):17–29.

30. Consroe P, Wolkin A. Cannabidiol-antiepileptic drug comparisons and interactions in experimentally induced seizures in rats. *J Pharmacol Exp Ther* 1977;201:26–32.

31. McGuire P, Jones P, Harvey I, et al. Morbid risk of schizophrenia for relatives of patients with cannabis-associated psychosis. *Schizophr Res* 1995;15:277–281.

32. Hézode C, Roudot-Thoraval F, Nguyen S, et al. Daily cannabis smoking as a risk factor for progression of fibrosis in chronic hepatitis C. *Hepatology* 2005;42:63–71.

33. Fisher BAC, Ghuran A, Vadamalai V, et al. Cardiovascular complications induced by cannabis smoking: a case report and review of the literature. *Emerg Med J* 2005;22:679–680.

34. Bari M, Battista N, Pirazzi V, et al. The manifold actions of endocannabinoids on female and male reproductive events. *Front Biosci* 2011;16:498–516.

35. Tyndale RF, Payne JI, Gerber AL, et al. The fatty acid amide hydrolase C385A (P129T) missense variant in cannabis users: studies of drug use and dependence in Caucasians. *Am J Med Genet B Neuropsychiatr Genet* 2007 (Jul 5);144B(5):660–666.

36. Di Forti M, Lyegbe C, Sallis H, et al. Confirmation that the AKT1 (rs2494732) genotype influences the risk of psychosis in cannabis users. *Biol Psychiatry* 2012;72:811–816.

37. Bhattacharyya S, Atakan Z, Martin-Santos R, et al. Preliminary report of biological basis of sensitivity to the effects of cannabis on psychosis: AKT1 and DAT1 genotype modulates the effects of delta-9-tetrahydrocannabinol on midbrain and striatal function. *Mol Psychiatry* 2012;17:1152–1155.

38. Hywel J, Williams MJ, Owen MC, et al. Is COMT a susceptibility gene for schizophrenia? *Schizophr Bull* 2007;33(3):635–641.

39. Cone EJ, Bigelow GE, Hermann ES, et al. Non-smoker exposure to secondhand cannabis smoke: I. Urine screening and confirmation results. *J Anal Toxicol* 2015 Jan–Feb;39(1):1–12.

40. Burns TL, Neck JR. Cannabinoid analgesia as a potential new therapeutic option in the treatment of persistent pain. *Ann Pharmacother* 2006;40:251–260.
41. Lynch ME, Campbell F. Cannabinoids for treatment of chronic non-cancer pain: a systematic review of randomized trials. *Br J Clin Pharmacol* 2011;72:735–744.
42. Neelakantan H, Tallarida RJ, Reichenbach ZW, et al. Distinct interactions of cannabidiol and morphine in three nociceptive behavioral models in mice. *Behav Pharmacol* 2015;26(3):304–314.
43. Johnson JR, Burnell-Nugent M, Lossignol D, et al. Multicenter, double-blind, randomized, placebo-controlled, parallel-group study of the efficacy, safety, and tolerability of THC:CBD extract and THC extract in patients with intractable cancer-related pain. *J Pain Symptom Manage* 2010;39:167–179.
44. Available at: http://www.medicalcannabis.com/cannabis-science/opioid-sparing/
45. Available at https://www.americanscientist.org/libraries/documents/200645104835_307.pdf
46. WebMD. Marinol: side effects. Available at: http://www.webmd.com/drugs/drug-9308-Marinol+Oral.aspx?
47. Available at: http://www.australasianscience.com.au/news/march-2014/herbal-cannabis-not-recommended-arthritis.htm
48. Issa MA, Narang S, Jamison RN, et al. The subjective psychoactive effects of oral dronabinol studied in a randomized, controlled crossover clinical trial for pain. *Clin J Pai.* 2014;30:472–478.
49. Wesnes KA, Annas P, Edgar C, et al. Nabilone produces marked impairments to cognitive function and changes in subjective state in healthy volunteers. *J Psychopharmacol* 2010;24:1659–1669.
50. Russo EB. The solution to the medical cannabis problem. In: Schatman ME, ed. *Ethical Issues in Chronic Pain Management.* New York: Informa Healthcare, 2007;165–194.
51. Available at: http://www.cdc.gov/nchs/data/databriefs/db166.pdf
52. Aggarwal SK, Pangarkar S, Carter GT, et al. Medical marijuana for failed back surgical syndrome: a viable option for pain control or an uncontrolled narcotic? *PM R* 2014;6:363–372.
53. Bachhuber MA, Saloner B, Cunningham CO, et al. Medical cannabis laws and opioid analgesic overdose mortality in the United States, 1999–2010. *JAMA Intern Med* 2014 Oct;174(10):1668–1673.
54. Available at: http://www.maps.org/research-archive/mmj/Abrams_2011_Cannabinoid_Opioid.pdf
55. Robson P. Therapeutic aspects of cannabis and cannabinoids. *Br J Psychiatry* 2001;178:107–115.
56. Crippa JA, Derenusson GN, Ferrari TB, et al. Neural basis of anxiolytic effects of cannabidiol (CBD) in generalized social anxiety disorder: a preliminary report. *J Psychopharmacol* 2011;25:121–130.

57. Ramikie TS, Nyilas R, Bluett RJ, et al. Multiple mechanistically distinct modes of endocannabinoid mobilization at central amygdala glutamatergic synapses. *Neuron* 2014 Mar 5; 81(5):1111–1125.

58. Bluett RJ, Gamble-George JC, Hermanson DJ, et al. Central anandamide deficiency predicts stress-induced anxiety: behavioral reversal through endocannabinoid augmentation. *Transl Psychiatry* 2014 Jul 8;4:e408.

59. Campos AC, Ortega Z, Palazuelos J, et al. The anxiolytic effect of cannabidiol on chronically stressed mice depends on hippocampal neurogenesis: involvement of the endocannabinoid system. *Int J Neuropsychopharmacol* 2013;16(6):1407–1419.

60. Bergamaschi MM, Queiroz RH, Chagas MH, et al. Cannabidiol reduces the anxiety induced by simulated public speaking in treatment-naïve social phobia patients. *Neuropsychopharmacol* 2011;36:1219–1226.

61. Zvolensky MJ, Cougle JR, Johnson KA, et al. Marijuana use and panic psychopathology among a representative sample of adults. *Exp Clin Psychopharmacol.* 2010 Apr; 18(2):129–134.

62. Cougle JR, Bonn-Miller MO, Vujanovic AA, et al. Posttraumatic stress disorder and cannabis use in a nationally representative sample. *Psychol Addict Behav.* 2011 Sep;25(3):554–558.

63. Neumeister A, Normandin MD, Pietrzak RH, et al. Elevated brain cannabinoid CB1 receptor availability in post-traumatic stress disorder: a positron emission tomography study. *Molecular Psychiatry* 2013;18:1034–1040.

64. Passie T, Emrich HM, Brandt SD, et al. Mitigation of post-traumatic stress symptoms by Cannabis resin: a review of the clinical and neurobiological evidence. *Drug Test Analy* 2012;4:649–659.

65. Roitman P, Mechoulam R, Cooper-Kazaz R, et al. Preliminary, open-label, pilot study of add-on oral Δ9-tetrahydrocannabinol in chronic post-traumatic stress disorder. *Clini Drug Invest* 2014; 34:587–591.

66. Available at: http://www.ptsd.va.gov/professional/co-occurring/ marijuana_use_ptsd_veterans.asp

67. Available at: http://www.medscape.com/viewarticle/836588

68. Das RK, Kamboj SK, Ramadas M, et al. Cannabidiol enhances consolidation of explicit fear extinction in humans. *Psychopharmacol (Berl)* 2013;226:781–792.

69. Leweke FM, Koethe D, Gerth CW, et al. Cannabidiol as an antipsychotic: a double-blind, controlled clinical trial on cannabidiol vs. amisulpride in acute schizophrenia. *Eur Psychiatry* 2007;22:S14.02.

70. Leweke FM, Piomelli D, Pahlisch F, et al. Cannabidiol enhances anandamide signaling and alleviates psychotic symptoms of schizophrenia. *Transl Psychiatry* 2012;20;2:e94.

71. Zuardi AW, Morais SL, Guimaraes FS, et al. Anti-psychotic effect of cannabidiol. *J Clin Psychiatry* 1995;56:485–486.

72. McLoughlin BC, Pushpa-Rajah JA, Gillies D, et al. Cannabis and schizophrenia. *Cochrane Database Syst Rev* 2014;10:CD004837.

73. Gates PJ, Albertella L, Copeland J. The effects of cannabinoid administration on sleep: a systematic review of human studies. *Sleep Med Rev* 2014;18:477–487.

74. Ashton H. Pharmacology and effects of cannabis: a brief review. *Br J Psychiatry* 2001;178:101–106.

75. Carlini EA, Cunha JM. Hypnotic and antiepileptic effects of cannabidiol. *J Clin Pharmacol* 1981;21(8–9 Suppl):417S–427S.

76. Nicholson AN, Turner C, Stone BM, et al. Effect of delta-9-tetrahydrocannabinol and cannabidiol on nocturnal sleep and early-morning behavior in young adults. *J Clin Psychopharmacol* 2004;24:305–313.

77. Izzo AA, Borrelli F, Capasso R, et al. Non-psychotropic plant cannabinoids: new therapeutic opportunities from an ancient herb. *Trends Pharmacol Sci* 2009;30:515–527.

78. Nagarkatti P, Pandey R, Rieder SA, et al. Cannabinoids as novel anti-inflammatory drugs. *Future Med Chem* 2009;1(7):1333–1349.

79. Collin C, Davies P, Mutiboko IK, et al. Sativex spasticity in MS study group: randomized controlled trial of cannabis-based medicine in spasticity caused by multiple sclerosis. *Eur J Neurol* 2007; 14:290–296.

80. Nguyen BM, Kim D, Bricker S, et al. Effect of marijuana use on outcomes in traumatic brain injury. *Am Surg* 2014 Oct; 80(10):979–983.

81. Ravikoff Allegretti J, Courtwright A, Lucci M, et al. Marijuana use patterns among patients with inflammatory bowel disease. *Inflamm Bowel Dis* 2013;19(13):2809–2814.

82. Cao C, Li Y, Liu H, et al. The potential therapeutic effects of THC on Alzheimer's disease. *J Alzheimers Dis* 2014;42(3):973–984.

83. Blake DR, Robson P, Ho M, et al. Preliminary assessment of the efficacy, tolerability and safety of a cannabis-based medicine (Sativex) in the treatment of pain caused by rheumatoid arthritis. *Rheumatology* 2006;45:50–52.

84. Alshaarawy O, Anthony JC. Cannabis smoking and serum C-reactive protein: a quantile regressions approach based on NHANES 2005–2010. *Drug Alcohol Depend* 2015 Feb 1;147:203–207.

85. Aqbal D, Abdallah A, Bolloso E, et al. The role of C-reactive protein in inflammatory bowel disease. *Georgetown University J of Health Sci* 2007;4(1).

86. De Filippis D, Esposito G, Cirillo C, et al. Cannabidiol reduces intestinal inflammation through the control of neuroimmune axis. *PLoS One* 2011;6(12):e28159.

87. Gracies JM, Nance P, Elovic E, et al. Traditional pharmacological treatments for spasticity. Part II: General and regional treatments. *Muscle Nerve Suppl* 1997;6:S92–120.

88. Pertwee RG. Cannabinoids and multiple sclerosis. *Pharmacol Ther* 2002 Aug;95(2):165–174.

89. Greenberg HS, Werness SA, Pugh JE, et al. Short-term effects of smoking marijuana on balance in patients with multiple sclerosis and normal volunteers. *Clin Pharm Ther* 1994;55:324–328.

90. Available at: http://www.mult-sclerosis.org/news/Sep2002/MedMJForMSSpasmsAndPain.html

91. Jody Corey-Bloom. Short-term effects of cannabis therapy on spasticity in multiple sclerosis. 2010 In: University of San Diego Health Sciences, Center for Medicinal Cannabis Research. *Report to the Legislature and Governor of the State of California presenting findings pursuant to SB847 which created the CMCR and provided state funding.* op. cit.

92. McCarthy DP, Richards MH, Miller SD. Mouse models of multiple sclerosis: experimental autoimmune encephalomyelitis and Theiler's virus-induced demyelinating disease. *Methods Mol Biol* 2012;900:381–401.

93. Foltin RW, Fischman MW, Byrne MF. Effects of smoked marijuana on food intake and body weight of humans living in a residential laboratory. *Appetite* 1988;11(1):1–14.

94. Le Strat Y, Le Foll B. Obesity and cannabis use: results from 2 representative national surveys. *Am J Epidemiol* 2011;174(8):929–933. First published online: August 24, 2011.

95. Struwe M, Kaempfer SH, Geiger CJ, et al. Effect of dronabinol on nutritional status in HIV infection. *Annals of Pharmacother 1993;* 27:827–831.

96. Beal JE, Olson R, Lefkowitz L, et al. Long-term efficacy and safety of dronabinol for acquired immunodeficiency syndrome-associated anorexia. *J Symptom Pain Manage 1997;*14:7–14.

97. Gross HA, Ebert MH, Faden VB, et al. A double-blind trial of delta-9-tetrahydrocannabinol in primary anorexia nervosa. *J Clin Psychopharmacol 1983;3:165–171.*

98. Todaro B. Cannabinoids in the treatment of chemotherapy-induced nausea and vomiting. *J Natl Compr Canc Netw* 2012 Apr; 10(4):487–492.

99. Ware MA, Daeninck P, Maida V. A review of nabilone in the treatment of chemotherapy-induced nausea and vomiting. *Ther Clin Risk Manag* 2008 Feb; 4(1):99–107.

100. ClinicalTrials.gov. A Study: Pure CBD as Single-Agent for Solid Tumor. NCT02255292. Available at: https://clinicaltrials.govict2/show/study/NCT02255292.Accessed December 21, 2014.

101. Watkins N. Insys' pharmaceutical CBD receives orphan drug designation for treatment of glioma. *Cannabis Pharma J* October 7, 2014. Available at: http://www.cannabispharmacyjournal.com/2014/10/07/insys-pharmaceuticalcbd-receives-orphan-drug-designation-for-treatment-of-glioma. Accessed January 4, 2015.

102. Torres S, Lorente M, Rodriguez-Fornes F, et al. A combined preclinical therapy of cannabinoids and temozolomide against glioma. *Mol Cancer Ther* 2011;10:90–103.

103. Available at: http://www.cancer.gov/cancertopics/pdq/cam/cannabis/healthprofessional/page4.

104. Kolodny RC, Masters WH, Kolodner RM, et al. Depression of plasma testosterone levels after chronic intensive marihuana use. *N Engl J Med* 1974;290(16):872–874.

105. Ramos JA, Bianco FJ. The role of cannabinoids in prostate cancer: basic science perspective and potential clinical applications. *Indian J Urol* 2012; 28(1): 9–14.

106. Armstrong JL, Hill DS, McKee CS, et al. Exploiting cannabinoid-induced cytotoxic autophagy to drive melanoma cell death. *J Investigative Dermatology* 2015;135:1629.1637.

107. Vara D, Salazar M, Olea-Herrero N, et al. Anti-tumoral action of cannabinoids on hepatocellular carcinoma: role of AMPK dependent activation of autophagy. *Cell Death Differ* 2011; 18(7):1099–111.

108. Nasser MW, Qamri Z, Deol YS, et al. Crosstalk between chemokine receptor CXCR4 and cannabinoid receptor CB2 in modulating breast cancer growth and invasion. *PLoS One* 2011;6 (9):e23901.

109. Shrivastava A, Kuzontkoski PM, Groopman JE, et al. Cannabidiol induces programmed cell death in breast cancer cells by coordinating the cross-talk between apoptosis and autophagy. *Mol Cancer Ther* 2011;10 (7):1161–1172.

110. Caffarel MM, Andradas C, Mira E, et al. Cannabinoids reduce ErbB2-driven breast cancer progression through Akt inhibition. *Mol Cancer* 2010;9:196.

111. McAllister SD, Murase R, Christian RT, et al. Pathways mediating the effects of cannabidiol on the reduction of breast cancer cell proliferation, invasion, and metastasis. *Breast Cancer Res Treat* 2011;129(1):37–47.

112. Aviello G, Romano B, Borrelli F, et al. Chemopreventive effect of the non-psychotropic phytocannabinoid cannabidiol on experimental colon cancer. *J Mol Med* 2012;90(8):925–934.

113. Romano B, Borrelli F, Pagano E, et al.: Inhibition of colon carcinogenesis by a standardized Cannabis sativa extract with high content of cannabidiol. *Phytomedicine* 2014;21(5):631–639.

114. Preet A, Ganju RK, Groopman JE. Delta-9-Tetrahydrocannabinol inhibits epithelial growth factor-induced lung cancer cell migration in vitro as well as its growth and metastasis in vivo. *Oncogene* 2008;27(3):339–346.

115. Mechoulam R, Carlini EA. Toward drugs derived from cannabis. *Naturwissenschaften* 1978;65:174–179.

116. Cilio MR, Thiele EA, Devinsky O. The case for assessing cannabidiol in epilepsy. *Epilepsia* 2014;55:787–790.

117. Devinsky O, Cilio MR, Cross H, et al. Cannabidiol: pharmacology and potential therapeutic role in epilepsy and other neuropsychiatric disorders. *Epilepsia* 2014;55:791–802.

118. Radke J. GW Pharmaceuticals provides update on their cannabidiol product to treat Dravet syndrome. Rare Disease Report, October 15, 2014. Available at: http://www.rarecir.comiarticies/GW-Pharmaceuticals-CannabidiolDravet-Syndrome. Accessed December 21, 2014.

119. Chagas MH, Zuardi AW, Tumas V, et al. Effects of cannabidiol in the treatment of patients with Parkinson's disease: an exploratory double-blind trial. *J Psychopharmacol* 2014;28:1088–1098.

120. Consroe P, Sandyk R, Snider SR. Open label evaluation of cannabidiol in dystonic movement disorders. *Int J Neurosci* 1986; 30:277–282.

121. Chagas MH, Eckeli AL, Zuardi AW, et al. Cannabidiol can improve complex sleep-related behaviours associated with rapid eye movement sleep behaviour disorder in Parkinson's disease patients: a case series. *J Clin Pharm Ther* 2014;39:564–566.

122. Naftali T, Bar-Lev Schleider L, Dotan I, et al. Cannabis induces a clinical response in patients with Crohn's disease: a prospective placebo-controlled study. *Clin Gastroenterol Hepatol* 2013; 11:1276–1280.

123. Morgan CJ, Das RK, Joye A, et al. Cannabidiol reduces cigarette consumption in tobacco smokers: preliminary findings. *Addict Behav* 2013;38:2433–2436.

124. American Psychiatric Association. *Diagnostic and Statistical Manual of Mental Disorders,5th Ed* (DSM5). Washington, DC: American Psychiatric Publishing, 2013.

125. Levin KH, Copersino ML, Heishman SJ, et al. Cannabis withdrawal symptoms in non-treatment-seeking adult cannabis smokers. *Drug Alcohol Depend* 2010;111:120–127.

126. Copersino ML, Boyd SJ, Tashkin DP, et al. Cannabis withdrawal among non-treatment-seeking adult cannabis users. *Am J Addict* 2006;15:8–14.

127. Mennes CE, Ben Abdallah A, Cottler LB. The reliability of self-reported cannabis abuse, dependence and withdrawal symptoms: multisite study of differences between general population and treatment groups. *Addict Behav* 2009;34:223–226.

128. Milin R, Manion I, Dare G, Walker S. Prospective assessment of cannabis withdrawal in adolescents with cannabis dependence: a pilot study. *J Am Acad Child Adolesc Psychiatry* 2008;47:174–178.

129. Crippa JA, Hallak JE, Machado-de-Sousa JP, et al. Cannabidiol for the treatment of cannabis withdrawal syndrome: a case report. *J Clin Pharm Ther* 2013;38:162–164.

130. Nussbaum AM, Thurstone C, McGarry L, et al. Use and diversion of medical marijuana among adults admitted to inpatient psychiatry. *Am J Drug Alcohol Abuse* 2015;41(2):166–172.

131. Moreira FA, Wotjak CT. Cannabinoids and anxiety. *Curr Top Behav Neurosci* 2010;2:429–450.

132. Niesink RJ, van Laar MW. Does cannabidiol protect against adverse psychological effects of THC? *Front Psychiatry* 2013;4:130.

133. Moran C. Depersonalization and agoraphobia associated with marijuana use. *Br J Med Psychol* 1986;59(Pt 2):187–196.

134. Reece AS. Chronic toxicology of cannabis. *Clin Toxicol* 2009; 47:517–524.

135. Price C, Hemmingsson T, Lewis G, et al. Cannabis and suicide: longitudinal study. *Br J Psychiatry* 2009;195:492–497.

136. Serafini G, Pompili M, Innamorati M, et al. Can cannabis increase the suicide risk in psychosis? A critical review. *Curr Pharm Des* 2012;18:5165–5187.

137. Hadland SE, Harris SK. Youth marijuana use: state of the science for the practicing clinician. *Curr Opin Pediatr* 2014;26:420–427.

138. Bally N, Zullino D, Aubry JM. Cannabis use and first manic episode. *J Affect Disord* 2014;165:103–108.

139. Volkow ND, Wang GJ, Telnag F, et al. Decreased dopamine brain reactivity in marijuana abusers is associated with negative emotionality and addiction severity. *Proc Natl Acad Sci U S A* 2014; 111(30);E3149–56.

140. Crippa JA, Zuardi AW, Martin-Santos R, et al. Cannabis and anxiety: a critical review of the evidence. *Hum Psychopharmacol* 2009; 24:515–523.

141. van Os J, Bak M, Hanssen M, et al. Cannabis use and psychosis: a longitudinal population-based study. *Am J Epidemiol* 2002; 156:319–327.

142. Ferdinand RF, Sondeijker F, Van Der Ende J, et al. Cannabis use predicts future psychotic symptoms, and vice versa. *Addiction* 2005;100:612–618.

143. McGrath J, Welham J, Scott J, et al. Association between cannabis use and psychosis-related outcomes using sibling pair analysis in a cohort of young adults. *Arch Gen Psychiatry* 2010;67:440–447.

144. Kuepper R, Van Os J, Lieb R, et al. Continued cannabis use and risk of incidence and persistence of psychotic symptoms: 10 year follow-up cohort study. *BMJ* 2011;342:d738.

145. Henquet C, Rosa A, Delespaul P, et al. COMT ValMet moderation of cannabis-induced psychosis: a momentary assessment study of "switching on" hallucinations in the flow of daily life. *Acta Psychiatr Scand* 2009;119:156–160.

146. Wu CS, Jew CP, Lu HC. Lasting impacts of prenatal cannabis exposure and the role of endogenous cannabinoids in the developing brain. *Future Neurol* 2011;6:459–480.

147. Karila L, Cazas O, Danel T, et al. Short- and long-term consequences of prenatal exposure to cannabis. *J Gynecol Obstet Biol Reprod* 2006;35:62–70.

148. Gray TR, Eiden RD, Leonard KE, et al. Identifying prenatal cannabis exposure and effects of concurrent tobacco exposure on neonatal growth. *Clin Chem* 2010;56:1442–1450.

149. American Academy of Pediatrics. Marijuana: a continuing concern for pediatricians. *Pediatrics* 1999;104:982–985.

150. Patton GC, Coffey C, Carlin JB, et al. Cannabis use and mental health in young people: cohort study. *BMJ* 2002;325:1195–1198.

151. Salomonsen-Sautel S, Sakai JT, Thurstone C, et al. Medical marijuana use among adolescents in substance abuse treatment. *J Am Acad Child Adolesc Psychiatry* 2012;51:694–702.

152. Grella CE, Rodriguez L, Kim T. Patterns of medical marijuana use among individuals sampled from medical marijuana dispensaries in Los Angeles. *J Psychoactive Drugs* 2014;46:263–272.

153. Fitzcharles MA, Clauw DJ, Ste-Marie PA, et al. The dilemma of medical marijuana use by rheumatology patients. *Arthritis Care Res* 2014;66:797–801.

The Future of Medical Cannabis

Predicting the future can often be frustrating and often wrong. However, I believe that several long-term secular trends can be followed to their most likely conclusion. Most of these trends have been alluded to or described throughout this book.

PREDICTION 1
Medical cannabis becomes broadly socially acceptable.

There is already a huge sea change underway in our society for acceptance of cannabis for medical use. Several polls have shown growing acceptance, well above 50 percent, among all age, gender, and race groups in the United States. Some polls suggest acceptance in the 80 percent range. With this acceptance, it will be easier for clinicians to recommend cannabis and not worry about their reputation among their patients who are not using cannabis. It will also be easier to add cannabis to treatment regimens in primary care practices.

PREDICTION 2
Medical cannabis will become legal in all of the states.

Medical cannabis—recreational, medical, or both—is now legal in more than half of the states. The trend toward legalization of medical cannabis has accelerated in the past few years. It is not unlikely for nearly all of the states to eventually pass medical cannabis legislation. In addition, cannabis may soon be moved from Schedule I to Schedule II or III. Either way, expect medical cannabis to be legal in the entire country within the next few years.

PREDICTION 3
CBD will be available over the counter throughout the United States.

CBD is already legal and available over the counter in more than half of the states. This CBD is extracted from hemp plants that are grown outside of the United States. With the greater appreciation of hemp for industrial purposes, large-scale hemp farms can be expected in the U.S., with ready availability of hemp and CBD oil. CBD is amazingly safe; it has no psychoactive effects and many measurable beneficial effects because of its anti-inflammatory and anti-anxiety properties. Expect CBD in oral or topical preparations to soon become readily available over the counter throughout the country.

PREDICTION 4
More and higher quality clinical studies of medical cannabis will be conducted.

The legalization of medical cannabis has made it much easier for doctors to conduct clinical studies, not just *in vitro* and *in vivo* basic research. More and higher quality clinical studies are already being conducted and the findings will be reported in the next few years. The number of conditions for which medical cannabis is proving efficacious is quickly expanding into neurodegenerative disorders such as Alzheimer's disease, autoimmune disorders, tumors, rheumatoid arthritis, and osteoarthritis. Expect the rate and diversity of clinical studies to expand in the next few years.

PREDICTION 5
Medical cannabis will become adjuvant therapy for more conditions.

With the forthcoming plethora of clinical studies on medical cannabis, it is likely that cannabis will be recommended treatment for an ever-expanding array of conditions and symptoms. If cannabis is moved out of Schedule I, clinicians will not have to pay attention to the quasi-scientific Qualifying Conditions list in each state, and can use it more liberally. However, it is expected that cannabis will remain adjuvant therapy directed at symptom control rather than primary therapy for a condition.

There will be more devices for potency testing.
As we gain an increasing understanding of the importance of CBD and THC potency and their ratio for therapeutic optimal effects, we should see more methods and devices for test- ing cannabis potency. In addition, with increasing popularity and demand for this type of technology for smartphones and home use, potency-testing devices should rapidly become less expensive.

There will be more use of smartphone apps and clinical application tools.
Along the lines of the new PotBot software, I expect the use of smartphone apps and clinical application tools available to cli- nicians to significantly help in selecting the type of cannabis medication, dosing, and route of delivery.

There will probably not be a major change in health insurance coverage.
This is difficult to prognosticate. Even if cannabis is put into a lower schedule, plant material such as oils and edibles, will, for the most part, not be FDA approved. In general, health insurance companies have to reimburse only for drugs that are both medi- cally necessary and FDA approved.

It is expected, and already happening, that some pharma- ceutical companies will produce a few proprietary cannabis products. Well-controlled formulations, such as mouth sprays, tinctures, oral films, and dermal patches, may make it through the stringent process of becoming FDA approved. However, most of the cannabis products in a typical dispensary will have to be purchased as an out-of-pocket expense by the patient.

The cost of caregiver services will probably remain a non- reimbursable expense. The caregiver's primary function is growing or obtaining cannabis for the patient. Since cannabis plants and most of the products at the dispensaries will still not be FDA approved, this function will still be outside of health insurance companies' purview.

PREDICTION 9
Cannabis products produced by pharmaceutical companies will become very popular.

With the expected FDA approval of Sativex and other FDA-approved cannabis patches and tinctures, it is expected that these will become very popular ways to administer cannabis. Unlike Marinol and Cesamet, these new products will be extracts of cannabis plants, with all of their THC, CBD, and terpenes present. The older pharmaceutical cannabis-products were analogues of THC, with significant adverse effects and lack of the clinically important entourage effect from the combination of THC with CBD and terpenes.

Clinicians will feel more comfortable prescribing these FDA-approved products. They will be available at regular pharmacies, without the need to send the patient to a cannabis dispensary. In addition, these medical cannabis products will be reimbursed by health insurance companies and will not carry the stigma that other cannabis products and paraphernalia have.

PREDICTION 10
Biosynthetic cannabinoids will be manufactured and made into pharmaceutical quality tablets, patches, and injections.

Current technology by various start-up companies will soon manufacture large quantities of inexpensive biosynthetic cannabinoids. Unlike the old synthetic cannabinoids from the 1980s, these biosynthetic cannabinoids are manufactured via fermented yeast methodologies and create true copies of the cannabinoids, not just similar analogues. In addition, this technology will allow—for the first time—large, inexpensive, quantities of the other cannabinoids to be created, such as cannabigerol (CBG), cannbicyclol (CBL), cannabichromene (CBC), and dozens of others. New effects and therapies will probably emanate from this easy availability of new medical molecules.

In addition, already patented techniques have created water-soluble cannabinoids, so that readily absorbed tablets, dermal patches, and injectable medications can be developed. These pharmaceutical quality medications will eventually be FDA approved and available in community pharmacies.

PREDICTION 11
Training of dispensary staff will improve, but eventually the role of dispensaries will diminish.

When the use of medical cannabis is legal in all 50 states under federal law, we should see greater uniformity in training and credentialing of dispensary staff, much like any of the other healing professions. Expertise in cultivation, extraction of cannabis plants, and production of edibles and tinctures will likewise require special training and certifications.

However, as FDA-approved cannabis medications become available and are reimbursed by health insurance, there will be a tendency away from obtaining medical cannabis at cannabis dispensaries toward getting it at regular pharmacies.

PREDICTION 12
Packaging and labeling of medical cannabis will improve.

There is already a huge push in states that have legalized medical cannabis to improve packaging and labeling. Many of the edibles and drinks are colorful and attractive to children; thus, child-proof packaging will be mandatory. In addition, many adults who are unfamiliar with edibles, or the cannabis dose in edibles, have been experiencing significant adverse psychoactive effects from too strong of a dose. Stricter control of dose and portion size is expected.

As discussed in a previous chapter, the potency labels on edibles and raw cannabis have been notoriously wrong. Fortunately, they have tended to overstate the amount of drug in the product. However, with improved state-mandated quality assurance programs and manufacturing processes, it is expected that these labels will become more accurate, similar to other medication labels.

PREDICTION 13
Banking and payment issues will be resolved.

Dispensaries should soon be able to use banks and take checks and credit cards. This will transform their current status as cash-only businesses. If cannabis is placed into a lower schedule or the federal government passes much-anticipated new banking regulations, then these decade old dispensaries will finally be able to conduct business normally. This will eradicate the challenges some patients face in needing to bring cash to the dispensary to buy their medication.

PREDICTION 14
Recreational cannabis will become legal in most states.

More states will legalize cannabis. This line of business will gradually grow separately from medical dispensaries. The sale of recreational cannabis will become more like that of alcoholic beverages, with popular brands of edibles, drinks, and high-THC and low-CBD cultivars of cannabis available on the open market. Freestanding cannabis stores or combined liquor/cannabis stores will become common.

PREDICTION 15
Clinician training on medical cannabis will become standard in medical school curricula.

This may just be wishful thinking, but I believe that in the next few years we can expect standard education modules on medical cannabis in medical school curricula. We can expect state medical boards to require several hours of continuing education on medical cannabis to make up for the historical lack of this education during training.

PREDICTION 16
Federal laws will change.

As of Fall 2015, there is a significant chance that federal legislation known as the Compassionate Access, Research Expansion, and Respect States Act of 2015 (CARERS) will be passed that will move cannabis from Schedule I to Schedule II. This one change in the law will significantly ease many of the logistical aspects of recommending cannabis for medical conditions. In addition, if this law is passed, then the clinician will be able to actually prescribe, not just recommend cannabis. In essence, it also would likely make the cost of cannabis-based medications reimbursable by health insurance.

Appendices

States Where Medical Marijuana is Legal and Restrictions

Summary Chart:

23 states and DC have enacted laws to legalize medical marijuana

State	Year Passed	How Passed (Yes Vote)	Possession Limit
1. Alaska	1998	Ballot Measure 8 (58%)	1 oz usable; 6 plants (3 mature, 3 immature)
2. Arizona	2010	Proposition 203 (50.13%)	2.5 oz usable; 0-12 plants
3. California	1996	Proposition 215 (56%)	8 oz usable; 6 mature or 12 immature plants
4. Colorado	2000	Ballot Amendment 20 (54%)	2 oz usable; 6 plants (3 mature, 3 immature)
5. Connecticut	2012	House Bill 5389 (96-51 H, 21-13 S)	One-month supply (exact amount to be determined)
6. DC	2010	Amendment Act B18-622 (13-0 vote)	2 oz dried; limits on other forms to be determined
7. Delaware	2011	Senate Bill 17 (27-14 H, 17-4 S)	6 oz usable
8. Hawaii	2000	Senate Bill 862 (32-18 H; 13-12 S)	4 oz usable; 7 plants
9. Illinois	2013	House Bill 1 (61-57 H; 35-21 S)	2.5 ounces of usable cannabis during a period of 14 days
10. Maine	1999	Ballot Question 2 (61%)	2.5 oz usable; 6 plants
11. Maryland	2014	House Bill 881 (125-11 H; 44-2 S)	30-day supply, amount to be determined

12. Massachusetts	2012	Ballot Question 3 (63%)	60-day supply for personal medical use
13. Michigan	2008	Proposal 1 (63%)	2.5 oz usable; 12 plants
14. Minnesota	2014	Senate Bill 2470 (46-16 S; 89-40 H)	30-day supply of non-smokable marijuana
15. Montana	2004	Initiative 148 (62%)	1 oz usable; 4 plants (mature); 12 seedlings
16. Nevada	2000	Ballot Question 9 (65%)	1 oz usable; 7 plants (3 mature, 4 immature)
17. New Hampshire	2013	House Bill 573 (284-66 H; 18-6 S)	Two ounces of usable cannabis during a 10-day period
18. New Jersey	2010	Senate Bill 119 (48-14 H; 25-13 S)	2 oz usable
19. New Mexico	2007	Senate Bill 523 (36-31 H; 32-3 S)	6 oz usable; 16 plants (4 mature, 12 immature)
20. New York	2014	Assembly Bill 6357 (117-13 A; 49-10 S)	30-day supply non-smokable marijuana
21. Oregon	1998	Ballot Measure 67 (55%)	24 oz usable; 24 plants (6 mature, 18 immature)
22. Rhode Island	2006	Senate Bill 0710 (52-10 H; 33-1 S)	2.5 oz usable; 12 plants
23. Vermont	2004	Senate Bill 76 (22-7) HB 645 (82-59)	2 oz usable; 9 plants (2 mature, 7 immature)
24. Washington	1998	Initiative 692 (59%)	24 oz usable; 15 plants

ProCon.org, "23 Legal Medical Marijuana States and DC: Laws, Fees, and Possession Limits." ProCon.org. 12 Nov. 2015 http://medicalmarijuana.procon.org/view.resource .php?resourceID=000881

Prototype of Recommendation Letter

DHS 9044 (4/05)

Medical Marijuana Program WRITTEN DOCUMENTATION OF PATIENT'S MEDICAL RECORDS (Please Print)

Note to Attending Physician: This is not a mandatory form. If used, this form will serve as written documentation from the attending physician, stating that the patient has been diagnosed with a serious medical condition and that the medical use of marijuana is appropriate. A copy of this form must be filed in the attending physician's medical records for the patient. If the patient chooses to apply for a Medical Marijuana Identification card through the county health department or its designee, the agency will call your office to verify the information contained on this form.

Attending physician name California medical license number

Service mailing address (number, street) Office telephone number

( )

City State ZIP code Office fax number

( )

Licensed by (check one):

Medical Board of California Osteopathic Medical Board of California

_____ is a patient under the medical care and supervision of the above Patient's name named physician who has diagnosed the patient with one or more of the following medical conditions:

1. Acquired Immune Deficiency Syndrome (AIDS) 2. Anorexia 3. Arthritis 4. Cachexia 5. Cancer 6. Chronic pain 7. Glaucoma 8. Migraine 9. Persistent muscle spasms, including, but not limited to, spasms associated with multiple sclerosis 10. Seizures, including, but not limited to, seizures associated with epilepsy 11. Severe nausea 12. Any other chronic or persistent medical symptom that either:

a. Substantially limits the ability of the person to conduct one or more major life activities as defined in the Americans with

   Disabilities Act of 1990. b. If not alleviated, may cause serious harm to the patient's safety or physical or mental health

ATTENDING PHYSICIAN STATEMENT:

This patient has been diagnosed with one or more of the foregoing medical conditions and the use of medical marijuana is appropriate.

Name of physician or physician staff completing this form Telephone number Date

Original—Patient Copy—Patient's File

Textbook Examination Questions

1. The ECS is involved with a variety of physiological processes, but not with:
   a. appetite
   b. pain sensation, mood, memory
   c. gastrointestinal functions
   d. muscle strength

2. All of the statements below are true, except:
   a. AEA is the principal ligand for CB1.
   b. 2-AG is the principal ligand of CB2.
   c. G Protein-Coupled Receptor 55 (GPR55) may soon be called CB3.
   d. Palmitoylethanolamide is the principal ligand of CB4.

3. CB1 is present in varying degrees in several structures within the brain, except:
   a. occipital cortex
   b. amygdala
   c. basal ganglia
   d. cerebellum

4. Which one of the following is not psychoactive?
   a. cannabidiol
   b. delta-9-tetrahydrocannabinol
   c. 11-hydroxy-delta 9-tetrahydrocannabinol
   d. delta-9-tetrahydrocannabinol

5. Which of the following is incorrect?

   a. Repeat exposure of cannabinoid receptors to ligands can lead to an increase in receptor density and coupling efficiency.
   b. Tolerance to the psychoactive effects of THC develop early, and the tolerance to the appetite stimulant effects take much longer.
   c. The two most well-studied phytocannabinoids are delta-9-tetrahydrocannabinol and cannabidiol.
   d. The available evidence shows that the density or coupling efficiency varies significantly in different centers of the brain.

6. Which of the following is incorrect?

   a. THC can aggravate psychosis.
   b. THC can aggravate anxiety.
   c. CBD can aggravate anxiety.
   d. CBD does not cause a psychological dependency syndrome.

7. Which of the following is incorrect?

   a. Marinol is a synthetic THC analogue.
   b. Sativex is a synthetic THC analogue.
   c. Cesamet is a synthetic THC analogue.
   d. JWH-018 is a synthetic THC analogue.

8. Which of the following is incorrect?

   a. Cannabis is superior clinically to synthetic THC for nausea and vomiting.
   b. Cannabis is superior clinically to synthetic THC for appetite stimulation.
   c. Sativex is superior clinically to cannabis for pain.
   d. Sativex is equivalent to cannabis clinically for anxiety.

9. Which is of the following is incorrect?

   a. It is legal to write a prescription for Marinol.
   b. It is legal to write a prescription for Charlotte's Web.
   c. Is is illegal to write a prescription for Sativex.
   d. It is illegal to write a prescription for cannabis edibles.

10. Which of the following is correct?

   a. Often decreasing the percentage of CBD will protect against the psychoactive side-effects of THC.
   b. The ratio of approximately 1:1 CBD to THC is the most studied, and appears to be a good start for most conditions.
   c. Psychoactive effects of CBD tend to lessen over time and with experience with titrating the medicine.
   d. Regarding CBD use, no neurologic, cardiac, psychiatric, sedation, or blood chemistry abnormalities have been identified.

11. Which of the following is not associated with a dependency syndrome?

   a. opioids
   b. THC
   c. CBD
   d. benzodiazepines

12. Studies have shown that patients who smoke cannabis usually use how much cannabis, divided over two to three doses per day?

   a. 0.3–1.0 grams per day
   b. 600–1500 grams per day
   c. 300–1000 grams per day
   d. 06.–1.5 grams per day

13. If a patient uses 1 gram per day of cannabis, which contains 20 percent THC, and the average joint is ½ gram, how many milligrams of THC are they inhaling with each joint?

    a. 200mg
    b. 50mg
    c. 100mg
    d. 500mg

14. How many average size joints are there in half an ounce of cannabis?

    a. 20
    b. 25
    c. 30
    d. 40

15. In general, which of the following routes of administration for cannabis-related medications results in the highest percent bioavailability of cannabinoids?

    a. oromucosal
    b. ingestion
    c. smoking
    d. vaporization

16. Which type of cannabis is recommended for treatment-resistant epilepsy?

    a. Low THC/High CBD
    b. High THC/Low CBD
    c. 1:1 THC/CBD
    d. Very low THC/High CBD

17. Smoking cannabis has been associated with which cancer?

    a. colon
    b. breast
    c. lung
    d. none of the above

18. Higher dose cannabis is not associated with which adverse effect?

    a. anxiety
    b. inhibition
    c. agitation
    d. hypertension

19. Which of the following statements regarding pharmacogenetic testing is incorrect?

    a. The Cytochrome P450 System, abbreviated CYP, is the most important system involved with cannabis metabolism in the body.
    b. If a CYP enzyme metabolizes a drug slowly, the drug stays a shorter time in the body.
    c. Because of the nature of genetic finger-printing, these tests are usually 99 percent sensitive and 99 percent specific when performed in high-quality laboratories.

20. Gene polymorphism may play a role in the link between THC and certain conditions. Choose the correct condition.

    a. schizophrenia
    b. depression
    c. insomnia
    d. eating disorders

21. Which route of administration for medical cannabis is not readily available?

    a. dermal patches
    b. vaporized
    c. injectable
    d. creams

22. Which of the following is incorrect?

    a. Very concentrated second-hand cannabis smoke in a closed environment may cause psychoactive or physiologic effects from the medication.
    b. Second-hand cannabis smoke can cause a positive urine drug test in certain extreme circumstances.
    c. Second-hand cannabis smoke has been associated with lung cancer.
    d. Second-hand cannabis smoke can aggravate respiratory conditions.

23. Which of the following is not a recommended form of cannabis-related medication?

    a. hashish
    b. edible candy
    c. THC enriched soda
    d. cannabis oil

24. Orally ingested cannabis results in which psychoactive metabolite?

    a. delta-9-THC
    b. delta-8-THC
    c. cannabidol
    d. 11-OH-THC

25. Which condition is cannabis not recommended for?

    a. fibromyalgia
    b. cachexia
    c. anorexia nervosa
    d. Dravet syndrome

26. For which type of pain is cannabis not recommended?

    a. chronic myofascial pain
    b. acute breakthrough cancer pain
    c. acute sprain/strain
    d. neuropathic pain

27. Which is the least common adverse effect for cannabis?

    a. cannabis dependence syndrome
    b. psychosis
    c. psychoactive effects
    d. hyperemesis syndrome

28. Which of the following is incorrect?

    a. THC can cause anxiety.
    b. THC can alleviate anxiety.
    c. CBD can cause anxiety.
    d. CBD can alleviate anxiety.

29. For which condition is adjunctive cannabis not recommended?

    a. THC for PTSD
    b. THC for panic disorder
    c. THC for insomnia
    d. CBD for schizophrenia

30. Which is the clinically superior medication for CINV?

    a. Sativex
    b. Cesamet
    c. cannabis 1:1 ratio
    d. 5-HT3 antagonist

31. Cannabis has antitumor effects through all of the following means, except?

    a. apoptosis
    b. inhibition of angiogenesis
    c. anti-inflammatory effects
    d. increasing circulating hormones

32. Studies support use of cannabis for all of the following cancers, except?

    a. melanoma
    b. prostate
    c. breast
    d. ovarian

33. According to the American Academy of Neurology review of the research from 1948 until 2013, cannabis may be useful for all of the following conditions, except?

   a. centrally-mediated pain
   b. multiple sclerosis
   c. epilepsy
   d. dyskinesias

34. Cannabis has not been shown to be useful for the treatment of which gastrointestinal condition?

   a. diarrhea
   b. nausea/vomiting
   c. irritable bowel syndrome
   d. inflammatory bowel disease

35. Which would be a possible medication to consider for cannabis dependence syndrome?

   a. CBD oil
   b. Sativex
   c. low-THC cannabis
   d. Cesamet

36. At this time, health insurance will not pay for which of the following medically necessary expenses?

   a. glass smoking bowl
   b. cannabis oil
   c. caregiver services
   d. all of the above

37. Cannabis has anti-inflammatory effects through all of the following, except?

   a. In the CNS via CB2 receptors found on microglial cells.
   b. CB2 receptors found on immune cells such as monocytes, macrophages, B cells, and T cells.
   c. CB2 receptors found on mast cells.
   d. In the CNS via CB2 and CB1 receptors found on cortical cells.

38. The antispasmodic effects of cannabis are recommended in the treatment of all of the following, except?

    a. acute muscle spasm from injury
    b. spasticity in MS
    c. spasticity in spinal cord injury
    d. spasticity in demyelinating disease

39. There are specific issues that the clinician should address with all of the following patient-types, except?

    a. pregnant women
    b. patients using chronic NSAIDs
    c. patients who work in hazardous environments
    d. elderly patients

40. In the review of peer-reviewed literature for the period 1990–2014 done by the organization ProCon.org, which was the least supported medical condition to treat symptoms with cannabis?

    a. multiple sclerosis
    b. bipolar disorder
    c. IBD
    d. rheumatoid arthritis

Textbook Exam Answers:

1.	d	11.	c	21.	c	31.	d
2.	d	12.	d	22.	c	32.	d
3.	a	13.	c	23.	d	33.	d
4.	a	14.	c	24.	d	34.	a
5.	a	15.	d	25.	c	35.	a
6.	c	16.	d	26.	c	36.	d
7.	b	17.	d	27.	d	37.	d
8.	c	18.	d	28.	c	38.	a
9.	b	19.	b	29.	b	39.	b
10.	b	20.	a	30.	d	40.	a

Index

blunt, 64
Boggs Act, 13
borneol, 20
brachial plexus injury, 77
breast cancer, 105–106
breastfeeding, 46, 49, 164
buds (flowers), 5–6, 18, 19,
54–58

C

C385A variant of FAAH, 137
California, 4, 14, 70, 72, 199
cannabichromene (CBC), 194
Canada, 74
Canadian Medical
Association, 74
cancer, 6, 71, 76, 77, 104–106
appetite stimulation and,
44, 98–99
breast, 105–106
chemotherapy-induced
nausea and vomiting
(CINV) and, 22, 40, 101,
103
colon, 106
glioblastoma multiforme,
106
glioma, 106
hepatocellular, 105
lung, 106
melanoma, 105
prostate cancer, 104
cannabidiol (CBD), xi, 35,
37–38, 114
amount in *Cannabis*
subspecies, 17, 18, 19
amount in new cultivars,
19

immunosuppression
caused by, 115
as over-the-counter
product, 63, 192
percentage of and
potency, 19–20
ratio of CBD and THC
and, 19, 22, 38, 114,
117–118
side effects from, 23, 115
cannabigerol (CBG), 39, 194
cannabinoid hyperemesis
syndrome, 102, 122–123
cannabinoid monitors, 149
cannabinoids. *see also
specific cannabinoids*
biosynthetic, xi, 194–195
cannabidiol (CBD). *see*
cannabiodiol (CBD)
phytocannabinoids, xiii,
21, 26, 28, 35–41
synthetic, xiii, 21, 22, 40,
43–51
tetrahydrocannabinol
(THC). *see*
tetrahydrocannabinol
(THC)
cannabinol (CBN), 28, 38, 39
cannabiodiol (CBD), 5, 28
cannabis, xi. *see also*
medical cannabis
19th-century laws
against, 13
20th century laws
against, 13, 14
history of use of, 11–15
home-grown, 53–54, 144
medical vs. recreational
use, 4, 118

reproductive system, affect
of medical cannabis on, 129
rheumatoid arthritis, 76, 80
Rhode Island, 73, 200

S

salvage patients, 163
Sativex (nabiximol), 24,
38–39, 50–51, 80, 118–119,
121, 123, 168, 194, xiii
Schedule I designation, 2, 5,
6, 14, 24
    attempts to change to
    Schedule II, 3, 15, 69, 71,
    128, 168
    limits on research due
    to, 76
schizophrenia, 76, 89–90,
138
seizure disorder, 71, 124
short-term memory, 122, 164
side-effects, 23–24, 83,
121–123
    cannabis dependence
    syndrome, 23, 114–115
    paranoia and anxiety, 86,
    115, 122
    psychoactive, 59, 62, 63,
    65, 82, 83, 84, 114, 116,
    117
    psychosis, 23, 76, 89–90,
    114–115, 122, 165
    ratio of CBD and THC
    and, 22
    screening for, 151,
    157–159
    short-term memory loss,
    122, 164
smartphone apps, 150, 193

smoked medical cannabis, 6,
55–56, 57–58, 76, 121
    bioavailability of, 123
    calculation of
    recommended dose, 20,
    63–65
    risk of lung cancer, 121,
    128–129
social anxiety disorder (SAD),
86
social stigma, 171, 191
spasticity, 71, 75, 96–97
special populations
    adolescents, 122, 156, 158,
    165
    geriatric patients, 46, 49,
    128, 166
    nursing mothers, 46, 164
    pediatric patients, 46, 49,
    128, 165
    pregnant women, 46, 49,
    128, 163–164
spice, 40
spinal cord injury, 77, 96
state law
    clinician training
    requirements, 72–74
    current status of, 70, 71,
    199–200
    legalized medical
    cannabis, 199–200
    medical cannabis
    legalization trends,
    191–192
    qualifying conditions,
    70–72
    recommendation letter
    requirements, 72
    on registered medical
    caregivers, 173